Healthy Tart!

Healthy Tart!

A healthy guide for women of all ages who want to look great and stay healthy regardless of all that 'Skinny Bitch' peer pressure.

By Trisha Stewart

© **2007 by Trisha Stewart**

Visit us on the web at:
www.HealthyTart.com
www.TrishaStewart.com
www.ChristinMcdowell.com

ISBN 978-0-9816846-4-2

Contents

Dedications

To Alison and Simon.

Life is either a daring adventure or nothing.

Helen Keller

Acknowledgements

Putting a book together with this amount of information is a team event. I would like to thank Mavis, Chris, Phil and the rest of the team for all their efforts and a special thanks to John Inman without whom, none of this would have happened.

Foreword

For 25 years I've helped improve the health and lifestyle choices of my clients. During that time I've seen improvements in medical science, an increase in available information relating various ailments to poor diet and obesity, more information about nutrition in the foods we eat and organic foods now readily available at major supermarkets. Yet, I am amazed...people in the western world do not seem to be getting healthier. In fact, the exact opposite seems to be occuring at alarming rates.

At my clinic in the Southwest of England, I've seen the steady deteriation of health, and worse 'health values'of the western world. How can we be bombarded with information and not be getting it? Half of the population struggles with the unhealthy desire to be skeleton thin "skinny bitches" nearly starving to death. And the rest seem to over induldge in every way possible, inviting ailments that should rarely affect us. That's why cancer, heart disease and diabetes among other diseases are now at epidemic proportions. It's insane!

Let's face it, most of us can never be (or don't want to be) super models. So why are we signing up to programs that we'll never achieve? Because most of the information you hear is misconstrued, too extreme or just plain wrong. Hear this! Too skinny is unhealthy! Too fat is unhealthy! So, where's the middle ground? Why can't we just be healthy, happy human beings who look normal? Let's get back to "Just Right"!

That's why I decided to write this book. I cannot stand by any longer and watch as people try to wade through a barrage of bad advice and misinformation. Believe it or not, there are too many people out there with vested interests in keeping you too skinny or too fat. They don't care if you're overweight or underweight, so long as you keep buying their products. Well, I say enough is enough!

That's why this book is about choices. It's about common sense. It's about having the right information...the truth. I want to see a change in attitudes towards our indulgences and I am one of the very few who have the experience, the knowledge and ability to educate and affect those changes.

Trisha Stewart, Devon UK, December 2007

Chapter 1

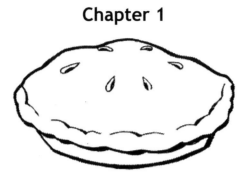

How in the "Health" are you?

What is a Healthy Tart?

Are you past the point of wanting to look like a malnourished super model? Have you come to the realization that being a size zero is neither an achievable nor a healthy goal? But, you still have the desire to be healthier, stronger, more fit...with more energy and vitality, right? You're tired of being tired...tired of knowing you're not living your best life? Then you have the mind set to become a Healthy Tart.

Let's just get it out there...a Healthy Tart is NOT a skinny bitch. If you're a Healthy Tart (or are ready to become one) you live in the real world with friends and family. You do not have militant attitudes about what you eat that you shove down other people's throats everywhere you go. You've never freaked out because someone sautéed your veggies in a skillet that once browned ground beef. You don't prefer packaged, processed vegan junk food to whole, natural foods – vegan or not. Sure, you may have tried a number of fad diets and schemes along the way...admit it, what woman hasn't used the 'grapefruit diet' at least once? But over time you've realized that health does not come in a pill or potion and that eating from only one food group just doesn't work. Finally, you understand that unless it is a long-term, livable lifestyle change...'diet' becomes another four-letter word you use in anger and frustration. Now you have (or are ready for) the TRUTH about food, cooking, supplements and exercise, and have achieved a balance that works consistently with your life. You just make the best decisions you can for you and your family when it comes to nutrition and lifestyle.

As a result, you are actually enjoying your life without over analyzing everything that crosses your lips. You have learned ways to shop, cook and eat healthy that fit your lifestyle and therefore you can actually stick with it. You don't condemn yourself if you eat a slice of cake at your cousin's wedding. You are healthy and have eliminated or reduced all or most medicines you used to take for various ailments. With your extra energy you're exercising in ways that are fun for you...that you actually look forward to!

Sound appealing? Sound right for someone in those "I'm really an adult and need to live that way" years as a sane, sensible and workable way to cut through the crap, forgo the fads and just get it done right? Then this book is for you. I'm going to outline the 10-step program that will convert you into the Healthy Tart you dream of becoming. Later we'll get into them in great detail, explaining the best approach, but here's a quick overview:

The 10 Steps

1. Clear the Decks: It's about getting rid of all the 'wrong' things you have in your kitchen, including out of date foods.

2. Equipment: Working juicers, sharp knives, healthy pots and pans...eating healthy starts with how you prepare your food.

3. Menu Planning: Waiting until the last minute to decide what to cook and eat is what gets most of us into trouble. Learn how to make menu planning easy.

4. Shopping: It's not just about a list of what to buy, but when to buy and how to make sure you're bringing home the good food.

5. Time Management: Like any new thing, you have to take time to make it work. This step is about staying on track even when you're at your busiest.

6. Goal Setting and Rewards: Without a target you will never know how you are doing. And, once you get there...you need to celebrate – the right way.

7. Move it and Lose it: This step is all about creating a working exercise plan for you and your lifestyle that actually gets results.

8. Detoxing: Do you need to perform a detoxifying cleanse? Why or why not? If so, how, when and what kind? Get the real truth on detox.

9. Body Treatments: While we're working on the inside, there are some key things you need to do to your outer-self as well.

10. Bringing it All Together: Prepping, cooking and juicing in the Healthy Tart way. A few reminders and basics to make it easier to get started and stay on track.

Through this journey you'll also learn that Healthy Tarts live in a place I call "Eden"...where all things are fresh, natural and good...life is fun and we have energy for the hard work and hard play that we love. Let me clarify that Eden is not about your faith or religion...it just represents that ideal place to live before chemicals, pollution, stress and worry muddied up our world and made living clean such a challenge.

Why I wrote the book!

Before I get into describing Eden, the 10-steps for getting there and how to claim and own your "Healthy Tartness" in vivid detail, I want to share with you a bit more about why I decided to write this book.

First, you are probably asking yourself...who the heck is Trisha Stewart? Why should I listen to this lady anyway? Great question, I'm glad you asked. And, by the way, being a healthy skeptic is a great trait of healthy tarts...but that's another book!

So, let me share with you a bit about my background and my own journey toward Eden. My interest in health and fitness began because I myself was overweight...even as a child. And, I watched people near and dear to me struggle with weight issues, but never make any long-term progress...every pound lost seemed to return with a friend or two. So, I made a decision to do things differently.

At the age of 23 I began working out in a gym and discovered I was altering the shape of my body...I became toned and in shape. That's where it all started for me because, for the first time in my life I actually felt good about myself. I was so excited that I wanted to help others get in shape and lose weight. So, I started working at different gyms. Then, I got really brave (or crazy) and ventured out on my own. I opened a state-of-the-art fitness center, which I ran for four years.

Now, as much as I loved my fitness center and my lifestyle, something still wasn't right. I struggled with fluctuating weight and digestive problems like bloating, constipation and PMS (this was nothing major but very irritating as it prevented me from being my best).

At the time, my nutritional knowledge was based on using proteins, carbs and fats for energy, muscle growth and general fitness...not for addressing illness or health challenges. So, I was eating meat, dairy, sugar and yeast...among other things. And, back then there was no one like me to talk to, so I didn't even know where to turn for advice.

I ended up consulting an open-minded homeopath. As he was just beginning his career, together we learned quite a lot and I took some major steps in my journey. After lots of reading and making small corrections here and there...I decided to become a vegetarian, eating just a bit of fish now and then (I have since given up the fish). It was amazing! My hormones balanced out, my digestion was fantastic, my weight reduced and – best of all - no bloating or constipation. I seemed very much in control of my body.

Okay, let's stop right here for a moment! In reading this, it all sounds rather simple, doesn't it? Just make a little change and poof...life is better. But, I can assure you it was NOT all that easy. It took me two years to sort myself out and there were some challenges and roadblocks along the way. The great thing is I've already done all the hard work for you and figured out the RIGHT way to make change happen. The 10-step program to becoming a Healthy Tart puts you in the fast lane towards optimum health. Plus, I'm available to guide you at every one of those steps. Now, before we delve into the steps, I need to share the rest of my journey with you.

Things seemed to be going great for me, but then tragedy hit. My wonderful 22 year-old son was lost at sea. He was working as a fisherman and apparently fell off the boat; no one realized he was missing for several hours. His body was never recovered. I'll never get over that loss; it affected my entire life. I truly thought I would never function as a normal being ever again. When it didn't seem it could any worse, three years later, my dear father was diagnosed with cancer.

He had already gone through surgery on his prostate and had a tumor removed from his bladder...he had been given the all clear. But 18 months later his cancer came back. By the time it was discovered, he was only given a few weeks to live. I felt so helpless...there was nothing I could do. I only understood fitness and health, not fighting cancer. Yet, it was these experiences and my father's insight that opened up the door to my current career. I was visiting him in the hospital when, referring to a dietician he admired, he looked at me and said, "You could do that." He was right and although at that time there was nothing I could do to help him, I just did not have the knowledge. So my path was clear and eventually, when my grief became less intense, I made it happen.

I studied massage, anatomy, physiology and nutrition...and became a certified teacher. So here I was, finally, a fully fledged complementary health practitioner. But, I needed more. I wanted to provide more accurate findings...and that meant more knowledge. I researched and came up with the BEST system for testing.

> The BEST (BioEnergetic Stress Testing) System represents the very latest in health screening technology. The System is fast, comprehensive and accurate. What is more, it is non-invasive and painless. There is no waiting around for the results - a detailed computer printout is available as soon as screening is completed, so both patient and practitioner know the situation immediately.
>
> *(see Fact File A for full description of the BEST system).*

It took me a year, with a trainer coming once a month to help me with my clients, for me to believe the system actually worked (not that I am cynic or anything!!!). I went on to train with an American college in Wales and that was where I tapped into the real depth of my knowledge. I learned about the BEST system, but moreover, I learned about disease. How it manifested...how the mind invaded the body...the problems with pollution...the connection of hormones and so much more - my passion was ignited! I had really found my niche and was able to learn, with great clinicians and Doctors, the truth about disease and how to regain great health. I had arrived!!

I have since worked with and helped hundreds of people with a countless array of health challenges. And it is because of my clients and their struggles and stories that are so important to my work that I decided to write this book. Too many times I've heard how their illnesses and maladies (diabetes, high blood pressure, IBS, colitis, Crohn's disease, arthritis, asthma, skin problems, overweight, underweight...you name it) just happened to them and it must be the "ravages" of aging or because they changed their job or had children or were bereaved.

They feel it's all but out of their control and there's nothing they could have done to prevent it. Not so!! The real truth is that the unhealthy lifestyle they have been leading for years has finally caught up with them. Our bodies will finally say...enough is enough! In fact, almost every health issue can be traced back to the type of lifestyle you lead and the choices you've made for years. Bottom line, things don't 'just happen'. Illnesses and health issues take time to manifest and my clients have been storing up years of bad choices to get them where they are.

I knew that my clients were not some unique 'sub-culture' of people. They weren't the only ones out there suffering and not realizing they had the power to make real changes to improve their lives. It was time someone got the truth out there for everyone! I know you're tired of hearing about the latest fad that seems to be just a pendulum swing of the last fad. You know what I'm talking about. *Eat low fat...eat low carb. Eat eggs...don't eat eggs...oh, wait – it's okay – eat eggs. Don't drink...have some wine. Don't eat fat...you need fat. Never eat sweets...chocolate is good for you. Take this pill, it blocks fats...no take this pill, it blocks carbs. Eat high protein...eat vegan...eat fast food and lose weight.* ARRRGHH!

It's no wonder people don't know what to buy and how to eat. And, keeping up with the latest craze can make you too tired to exercise (let alone figure out which exercises are right for you). So, there you are unsure if you should eat by your blood type, zodiac sign or shoe size! It's enough to make anyone say, "Why bother?"   But, if you're reading this book...you know there are some real answers out there and you're looking for them. You really want to start living your best life. You want to become a Healthy Tart. And, I want to help. So, really I'm writing this book for YOU...to tell you the truth.

Let me say this now...it's never too late to start. Don't worry, I've heard all the reasons and excuses that have kept you from achieving health success before, and can address them all. So, no matter where you are, whatever level of fitness, you can get closer to Eden and work your way towards becoming a Healthy Tart. I'm here to help you make that happen and this book is just the beginning to tapping into what you can achieve. Beyond this book, there's ongoing support and resources on my website that will be there as you continue your journey toward real, lasting health...toward Eden.

My Philosophy
You've probably started to pick up on my philosophy already...the way I approach health and life. And, by the end of this book, you'll know how that philosophy applies to every detail of your lifestyle...from what goes in to your body to how you use it to how you get rid of it. Yes, I will speak in vivid detail about digestion and elimination as it really is the core of good health. But, let me sum up for you my overall philosophy...what I like to call my "Back to Eden Attitude".

The "Back to Eden Attitude"
Through the ancient 'hunter/gatherer' approach to daily life of eating what one   could catch and gather, what was in season, grown, ripened by the natural sunlight and washed by

clean rainwater...all adapted for today's workaday world...I help people not just survive, but thrive. By creating a program that encourages total wellness at a personalized pace, they regain control of their lives and the power within them to be strong, fit, vibrant and healthy. In essence my work is about educating people to live naturally, allowing normal body functions, increased mental agility and a fulfilled happy life in harmony with mind, body and spirit.

Chapter 2

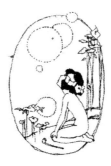

The Garden of Eden *(Where Healthy Tarts Live & Thrive)*

It's no big surprise that we don't live in idyllic surroundings, but wouldn't it be great if we could? Imagine what it would be like to live in an environment where everything worked to and for the greater benefit...the greater good. Do you think it was ever like that? To hear our more seasoned citizens speak, things were certainly better in the "good old days." In fact, you may be approaching 'that certain age' where you fondly remember the simpler times of your past. You may have already uttered that phrase (unless you caught yourself), "Well, when I was younger..."

Is there any truth to it? Were things better in the 'good old days'? Well, to a certain extent, yes...things were better...if we go way back...to the Garden of Eden. Now, let me clarify that what I'm referring to is not a religious or faith-based Eden...I'm using the idea of "Eden" as the idyllic place where life was easy, health was a given and there weren't so many distractions, obstacles and dangers to challenge our living and thriving. In other words, it's a place where every woman is a Healthy Tart and being and maintaining that health seems as natural as breathing. What would this Eden be like?

Imagine a gorgeous sunny day...not too hot, but just right. You walk outside to enjoy the sunshine...without the worries about skin cancer from harmful rays. And, as you look up into the bright blue sky you see a few white clouds wisp by, but that's it. Off into the distance there is nothing but more clear skies...no haze, no smog. You breathe deep knowing you're inhaling fresh, clean air. As you walk along you take a drink from a bottle of water you've brought with you...filled directly from your own tap. Of course, if you wanted, you could also drink clean, pure water from a nearby stream or fountain. There is no need for filters, pumps or sanitizers...all accessible water is just naturally clean.

You stop at a local farmer's market to select from an abundance of fresh fruits, vegetables, nuts and more. All grown naturally and locally, and with so much variety you can't begin to try everything that catches your eye. While you pick produce, breads and grains for the week, you're able to sample any and everything right on the spot. Since there are no pesticides or chemicals used, the most you have to do is brush off a bit of natural dirt before taking a bite of whatever catches your eye.

Back home you begin to prepare a meal with all your fresh ingredients. No pre-packaged, readymade or processed foods...just healthy, nutritious and good tasting dishes to savor and enjoy with your family and friends. That's right...everyone sits down at the table at the same time because spending time together is not only a priority, but an expected daily occurrence. Any minor stresses of the day are easily set aside as you all focus on enjoying each other's company.

After a glorious meal, everyone heads out for a brisk walk...exercise being something that you look forward to and enjoy. Your steady diet of nutritious foods, regular exercise and good company means you and your family are always healthy. No allergies, illnesses or ailments slow you down as you make the most out of every day living and thriving with vitality.

That sounds pretty good, doesn't it? If we could create this Eden for you and you moved there...you would naturally thrive, enjoy life more and be happier and healthier...it would be easy...almost effortless. But, I know that's not your everyday world. There are so many things you have to worry about, deal with, accept or give up on altogether. Sometimes it feels like a major accomplishment to just get through the day, right? So, what exactly does your real world look like?

The alarm wakes you from a restless sleep and you struggle to get your feet onto the floor. Already behind schedule you rush around to get yourself (and anyone else) in the house ready to leave for the day. A quick cup of coffee and a packaged breakfast bar of some sort – filled with more chemicals and preservatives than nutrition – a substitute for breakfast. You jump into your car and you're off to fight overwhelming traffic get yourself to work...or your kids to school...or the dog to the groomers...whatever is on your list first thing in the morning.

The weather forecast says sunny, but all you see when you look out your windshield is a haze of smog and pollution that make you wonder if you should be breathing air you can actually 'see.' Of course, if you have kids, there was no time to fix them a healthy lunch. So you dole out money they can use to buy what you know will end up being too many chips, snacks and other junk food, but it's better than nothing – you hope.

Arriving at your office, or your first appointment, you already feel defeated as you face a mountain of work, chores and errands that seem overwhelming. Your day is spent rushing from meeting to phone call to checking emails to an appointment (that you're late for because of traffic...again).

And, that 'to do' list just seems to get longer. Lunch (remember there was no time to fix something healthy from home) is a bottle of water that may or may not be any better for you than plain tap water and a burger someone brought back for you from a lunch run or something you grabbed at the convenient mart while you gassed up your car. Then it's time to pick up the kids...or the dog from the groomers...or the dry cleaning...oh and don't forget you need to stop get some grocery shopping done.

Fighting traffic the entire way you manage to collect and pick up whatever...or whomever...you were supposed to and then stop by the grocery store for the week's supplies. You pass by the fresh produce as you never have time to cook those things before they go bad. Instead, because time is tight, you buy frozen and canned vegetables, a few readymade meals and frozen pizzas, some processed preservative laden sandwich meat and a few boxes of sweetened cereal or some other quick breakfast food.

As you get back into the car, you realize that you are so tired the thought of even 'nuking something in the microwave' sounds like a lot of effort. Plus, you're getting cranky (low blood sugar), so you pull through a fast food drive-thru and order something that passes for dinner. Exhausted, you arrive home and collapse on the sofa for a few minutes of rest. Then, a few rounds of laundry or some other housekeeping chore before you fall into bed. You hope housework really does count as exercise, because that's the only physical activity you've had in months. Now, you're already worrying about tomorrow's schedule and that means another restless night.

Oh yes, some of those descriptions you recognize – don't you? Probably more than you'd like to admit with the stress, too much to do, no time for self and more. In fact, these days it's not surprising that some of you may be thinking...I know something I'm doing...or not doing...is going to kill me, they just haven't figured out what it is yet.

So, if this is the world you live in and it seems to be just getting worse, why would I describe some Eden-like place where you can thrive? Why describe some place that's so far removed from reality that it can never exist? Because...at least on some level...it can exist.

The Healthy Tart approach to life takes you step by step back to an Eden-like existence that also factors in and works with the real world where you work and play. I understand that we live in a modern society and some of the things that are keeping us from Eden are modern conveniences that you're just not going to give up. And perhaps you can't give up without major difficulty. So rest assured I don't expect you to move out into the wilderness with no electricity, surviving on berries and twigs! What I've created for Healthy Tarts is a way to claim your corner of Eden amid the workaday real world. I admit that following this program won't put an end to the pollution in our air, but it will ensure your body can deal more efficiently with all that external pollution...and that's a major accomplishment!

Now, here's where my approach differs from some of the many 'quick-fix' plans and program you've seen on TV and read about in books. I'm not promising you success overnight – or even in 30 days. I am talking about lifestyle changes you'll be able to live with – and thrive on – forever. So, I encourage slow changes, what I call 'one percent changes'. That is unless there's a major health risk involved and drastic measures are needed. If that's the case, a visit to www.TrishaStewart.com is in order to get more personalized support for your health challenge.

So, what are 'one percent changes'? They are incremental changes or shifts in your habits that are doable and can be entrenched in your life like brushing your teeth. You've already tried the 180-degree turnaround...maybe more than once. And what happened? You started out great, but because there were so many new things to handle and get used to, it was difficult to keep it up. The "real world" snuck in and your busy schedule took over. Before you knew it, you were right back where you started and not only had you not maintained the healthy changes you had hoped for, you felt like a bit of a failure. Well, I want to set you up for success...not failure. It's better to make one small change and keep it than to try for ten big changes and let them all go. That's why I've created the 10-step program...a way to systematically introduce changes to your life. And, my 30-day plan is a subtle introduction to eating, juicing and exercising for optimum health.

And, the great thing is that if you need more guidance on getting started, customizing your plan due to health challenges or sticking with it for the long-term...there's support, information and coaching available through my website. So, just log onto www.TrishaStewart.com and change your life...one percent at a time.

Chapter 3

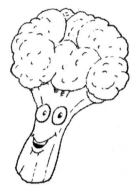

It's what's on the inside that counts

You've heard it before...you are what you eat...and it's true, but why? Great question! It goes beyond the fact that if you eat fattening foods, you'll be overweight. It's what the food you eat does - or doesn't do - to help your body function. Here's the deal – I believe most health problems are linked to poor diet, pollution and stress...conditions like migraine headaches, asthma, depression and more.

Most people don't really understand how our bodies work and what's going on when it doesn't work. Do you really think that a headache is caused by a lack of pain reliever in the body? No, but that's how most people treat a headache...often ignoring the root cause of what's really going on. Here's a hint...it's very often connected to your diet. I can't tell you how many clients I have who come to me thinking their bodies are really no more than a vehicle to carry their heads around...I'm serious! But there has never been anything invented, grown or produced that is so wonderful, so apparently simple, yet so complicated when it is abused. And, part of being a Healthy Tart living thriving in Eden is that your body is running and working at its best from the inside out. But, telling you what foods to eat and how to exercise is only part of the equation (and we'll be getting to that soon)...you need to understand what's going on inside...your digestive, immune and endocrine (hormonal) systems.

DIGESTIVE SYSTEM

For me this is where health begins or deteriorates. Your digestive system is more than your stomach and intestines; it also includes your kidneys, liver and pancreas. But, let's get down to it...it's about the end result...that's right – your bowel health. You CANNOT be seriously healthy if your bowels are not acting in the way they should.

Now I'm sure this is not a topic you like to discuss...people get very quiet about their bowels, but I believe it's actually appropriate dinner conversation! Okay, there is a time and place for everything, but it's an absolutely normal and vital function. And, when I turn up as a dinner guest (and people know who I am) they love to turn the conversation to their gut and bowel functions. That's probably because they know I'll directly ask the question, "How are your bowels?" So, beware if you invite me for dinner!

Why am I so interested in your bowel movements?
Because bowel disorders are often a direct link to many ailments and diseases.

Most bowel disorders are some form of constipation. Do you realize that your bowels need to evacuate more than once every day? What do you think will happen to the putrefied waste in your body if it cannot escape? Think about it! Constipation is linked to all manner of stomach disorders, parasites, Candida, diverticulitis, colitis, indigestion, stomach cramps, backache and any other inflammatory bowel condition.

But, all too often people do not have healthy bowel movements...and don't even know it. It often happens to the elderly and they believe it's just a part of aging. It isn't! Constipation in the elderly is usually linked to lack of exercise, little or no water intake, poor diet and overuse of prescription drugs. The unfortunate result is that if there is too much in the system and it's not coming out in a bowel movement, their bodies will regurgitate the contents of what should be going through the colon...poo!!! Yes, this is true. And, it has also been reported that children today are so constipated through poor diet and lack of exercise they too are regurgitating the contents of the colon.

Not only is the thought of this not pleasant, but it's very detrimental to your health. You see, the digestive system has various "one way" valves whereby foods, partially or digested, pass through the valves but cannot or at least should not come back up due to the very clever design. But, if waste is trying to come back up that is a hell of a lot of pressure pushing on your system! No wonder constipation or poor bowel movements can throw your entire body off kilter.

Okay, you get it, right? The end result is really where it starts. If you don't have a working, healthy digestive system...there is NO WAY that you can be a healthy person...or a Healthy Tart! But don't panic! Even if you're not in 'digestive shape' right now, you can get there with The 10 Steps to Eden. The 30-day plan I outline at the end of the book is a great starting point for everyone, but those with any digestive issues will notice measurable benefits right away.

IMMUNE SYSTEM

Your amazing body is very interlinked...one system supporting and working with the other. Your digestive and immune systems are no exception. So, please understand this...a weakened digestive system affects your immune system. Bottom line...that means not eating right leads to a bowel disorder that weakens the immune system and before you know it...you've got a chronic disease to deal with on top of poor digestion. But, you probably don't know they're related.

Well, of course, now you do, don't you? You've probably been hearing more and more about your immune system...but what exactly does it do?

The immune system is like the front line...a network of cells and organs that defend the body against microbes or tiny organisms including bacteria, viruses, parasites and fungi. In other words, our immune systems helps keep us healthy by fighting back against the onslaught of illnesses, infections and diseases we come in contact with every day. It either keeps them out or kills them off...when it's working correctly. When your immune system is weakened things slip through the cracks. On a minor level that's when you get overtired and have a cold. On a grander scale, a perpetually weak immune system is tied to diseases including chronic fatigue, fibromyalgia and more. For you "Detail Divas", check out Fact File D for a complete rundown of the technical side of your immune system.

Food allergies are also connected to the immune system. When your body is over-stimulated by a certain food or allergen...your immune system attacks the body. Without getting too complicated, what happens is your body creates antibodies which react to the food/allergen. This causes the immune system to release histamines and other chemicals that causes an 'allergic' reaction. Symptoms can be as mild as bloating, diarrhea, constipation...or more severe including skin rashes, swelling of the throat, face or tongue, to loss of consciousness and even death.

But, here's the truth...most people do NOT have food allergies...they have food intolerances due to poor digestive function. So, what you actually feel is more often than not the result of a compromised digestive system, which will cause an immune response as there is a mass of lymphoid tissue in your gut. It can be the result of eating a certain food, combination of foods or even a particular ingredient in a food. Symptoms of food intolerances include headaches, nausea, bloating, diarrhea, skin irritations, blocked sinuses, chronic fatigue, fibromyalgia, period pain, menopausal symptoms and more.

The tricky part is they can occur anytime from right after eating to up to 72 hours later. So, it can be very difficult to detect which particular food or combination of foods that has been eaten that has caused your symptom. Yet, while tracking down which specific food you may be intolerant to, treating it is very doable. The good news is that depending on severity of condition, length of time suffered, a change of diet, supplementation and healing remedies are all that is needed to restore good health and vitality.

HORMONAL (ENDOCRINE) SYSTEM

We all have them...and we're all affected by them. But, I bet you thought hormones only dealt with sex and your mood didn't you? Not so! There are many hormones, each with their own special messenger function - flying through the blood system to deliver needed information or signals.

The endocrine system is probably one of the most ignored systems in the body, but mostly because people don't understand what it does. This collection of glands is often called the communication system - or the chemical system. I'm sure you've heard people talk about meeting someone and that the "chemistry" just felt right. Well, there really is an automatic, physical reaction when you meet someone you're attracted to. The thought process of your brain sends a signal to your hormonal system when you feel a connection with someone. That's the way the endocrine system works...sending chemical signals throughout the body to help it operate, function and survive.

So, what kind of signals do your hormones send? I mean besides that 'chemistry' thing we've all experienced a time or two (and would like to experience even more often, I'm sure)! It's more complicated and detailed than I will go into here, but everything from your 'fight or flight' response to blood sugar levels to how you metabolize and use food as fuel are all results of the messages your hormones send throughout your body. For a deeper picture into your endocrine system read Fact File E.

So, hormones are much more than our sexuality and mood indicators. We need these chemical messengers to keep our bodies operating at peak potential! Now, it's hopefully a bit clearer how inter-connected the digestive, immune and endocrine systems are, and more importantly, how greatly influenced their performance is by what we eat.

Chapter 4

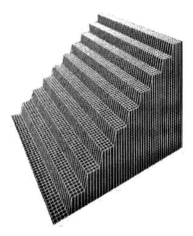

Ten Steps to Eden

Are you ready? Let's get you started on your own personal road to Eden where you can live and thrive as a Healthy Tart. I'll be upfront and say...this won't be easy! There, I've said it. But, let me counter with the reality that it won't be impossible either. In the steps I've created there are no magic pills, shakes or potions that will turn you into a Healthy Tart overnight. But, remember that it took you years to get your body in the state it's in...good, bad or ugly...and you know who (or where) you are. So, let's face this together...it's going to take some time to get back to your ideal self. But, not to worry...you're not in this alone. Not only do I outline all the steps and explain them in detail, I've provided a 30-day launching pad, shopping lists, menus and recipes to ease your transition. Plus, my website is a 24-hour/seven days a week resource for you for support, encouragement, answers and more. But, we'll get to all of that later. Now it's time to read over these life changing steps and what's involved.

Okay, I know you've heard this before, but please read ALL the steps before you get started. You need to understand the entire program before you jump into the first step. And, of course, as you read along you'll have questions...some of which will be answered in subsequent steps, in my Details Diva Appendices. Believe me, with my years of seeing patients, I have been asked every question imaginable...so I'm confident I've answered almost everything you can think of. However, if I've missed something...you can always email me. I want you to have the information and tools you need to succeed. And what about obstacles...things that get in the way when we try any new lifestyle program or regime? They're out there. But, I've helped people face them all and have dedicated an entire chapter to the most common challenges. So, let's get cracking!

TEN STEPS TO EDEN
The Home of Healthy Tarts

1. **CLEAR THE DECKS**
   Out with the old...in with the new (and better)...getting your kitchen ready

2. **THE RIGHT TOOLS FOR THE RIGHT JOB**
   The equipment you need to succeed and what 'jobs' you'll be doing

3. **MENU PLANNING**
   Prior planning increases success and makes life sane

4. **SHOP 'TIL' YOU DROP**
   What to buy, when to buy and how to stock your kitchen

5. **TART TIME MANAGEMENT**
   How to be a Healthy Tart on a busy schedule

6. **GOAL SETTING & REWARDS**
   Doing it for yourself and celebrating your victories

7. **MOVE IT AND LOSE IT**
   Exercise, posture and movement

8. **DETOX OR NOT-DETOX**
   The truth about detox cleanses

9. **BODY TREATMENTS**
   Taking care of the outside matters

10. **BRINGING IT ALL TOGETHER**
    Prep and Cooking for the Healthy Tart

Step 1. CLEAR THE DECKS
Out with the old...in with the new

Whether you know it or not...a lot of the food in your kitchen is not fit to eat. Of course there's the obvious stuff (candies, cookies chips and the like), but it goes much deeper than you think. Some of the very items you believe are healthy may need to get tossed into the rubbish. Don't panic! After you rid your kitchen of the 'old'...you'll have plenty of room for the beautiful 'new'. But, that's Step 4...so be patient.

First, you need to throw out all of your out of date dried ingredients. Apart from just tasting old and stale, they're likely covered in molds (see **Fact File P: How to Handle & Avoid Moldy Food**). That's right...molds! The tricky thing about mold like this is you can't see them...but trust me, it's there. So, what are the dried ingredients you should toss out? If any of the following items have been in your cupboard for more than six months, then throw it out and get fresh: Nuts, lentils, dried beans, oats, flour, pasta, rice, millet, barley, any grains or cereals... you name it...I am sure it will be out of date.

Next, head for the freezer and immediately throw out anything that's been in there for more than six months. You know what I'm talking about...that half bag of frozen vegetables, the forgotten tub of ice cream that now has a layer of ice on it, the opened bag of french fries, that piece of meat you can no longer recognize (is that chicken or beef?), the left over something that has no name, frozen pastries, ancient frozen orange juice...even the stale ice cubes! The list could go on for a number of pages, but you get the idea. If it's been in your freezer for half a year...it does NOT need to go into your mouth. THROW IT OUT!

Okay, time to hit the fridge. This can be scary, but be brave...bend over and pull out that bottom crisper drawer. You know the one that's supposed to keep produce nice and fresh (hence the name 'crisper drawer'). You know what's there...those sad, tired, old and withered vegetables that you were going to cook but never got around to it. Oops, you forgot about the nice cucumber, didn't you? If it looks like a science experiment or is limp and rubbery...it's out. You may need to get some gloves and a gas mask...but do it. It only hurts a little bit. Okay, now before you close the door...move up to the other shelves. Any leftovers you can no longer recognize need to be pitched out. Doesn't matter if it's Aunt Hilda's special soup or Teriyaki chicken from your favorite restaurant...if it's more than a couple of days old...let it go. Add to that any sad looking jars with bits of condiments...a touch of mayonnaise, a dab of relish, a few maraschino cherries, cocktail onions or olives...why do we have those anyway? Oh, you're probably thinking...my refrigerator is so bare...it may even look a little sad. Not to worry...you've made room for all the lovely new foods that are going to be in there very soon.

Next hit the cookie jars, snack baskets and candy bowls to clear out and give away any cookies, cakes, chocolates or other sweet temptations. Remove them from your sight...it takes a while, but out of sight really does lead to out of mind with sweet snacks. Okay – okay, if they belong to another member of the family, you might get in big trouble for giving away their favorite decadent pleasure. So, for now put them in a section of the kitchen just for them. Be ready though, because once they see how you progress, it won't be long before they won't want to eat them either!!

What else needs to go? Here's a quick list of items to ban from your kitchen:

o   Microwave ready meals...including those so-called healthy or diet dinners

o   Hydrogenated margarine and butter

o   Low fat dressings...remember low fat here means probably full of sugar

o   Fruit yogurt...again the label says 'low fat' but it possibly translates into 'loadsa sugar'!

o   Processed lunch meat and cheese for sandwiches

o   Sodas or soft drinks (even the diet ones)

o   Chemical laden beer

o   Sulphite rich non-organic wine

o   Diet shakes (ready-made or powdered)

So, are you beginning to see what to remove and throw out? Great! Now, if you still have a few items you're not sure about...check out the shopping list at the end of the book and you'll have a perfect list of the great foods you SHOULD have in your kitchen. And, if you're like me and want to know more of the whys behind getting rid of some of these processed, packaged and pumped up foods...see Chapter Six, *The Good, the Bad and the Very Ugly*

After you've removed all the bad, unhealthy, old, stale and processed foods, you also need to prepare your cooking areas. Sure you wipe things down on a daily basis, but now is the time for a deep clean. Please...use a natural cleaning product...you do not want to introduce more chemicals into your world. Scrub and disinfect the counter tops, pull out the burners on the stove and make them sparkle and remove all the baked on 'stuff' out of the oven...this may take some real elbow grease, but it's worth it. Make your cooking and preparing spaces ready for your new regime. It's out with the old...so you can bring in the new! Now, what about all your pots, pans and processors? Let's move on to Step 2!

Step 2. THE RIGHT TOOLS FOR THE RIGHT JOB
The equipment you need to succeed

You've heard it said that the right tool for the right job makes all the difference in the world. Well, that's just as true in the kitchen as it is on the job site. So, let's take a look at what kitchen equipment you need and what you don't need...and why. There may be a few new ideas or concepts in here...but I'll walk you through it. Don't forget to check out our Detail Divas Appendices that offer more information on certain topics.

Ahhh...the power of Juice
If it's not already, juicing is going to be a big part of your life. That means you need a juicer and/or smoothie maker...something that can turn fresh fruits and vegetables into wonderful health-filled drinks. If you already have one...make sure it's clean and ready to use...check the crevices and crannies for old, crusty food that's harboring mold and bacteria. If you don't have a juicer or smoothie maker...it's time to go shopping! Remember, this is not a luxury...this is a vital piece of equipment for your long-term health...in other words an investment. While you don't have to purchase the most expensive model, be sure to get a reliable product that won't break down after one month's regular use. Look for one that has a large opening, to take

whole or large chunks of fruits and veggies. I prefer a masticating style as this process is like chewing the produce; extraction is slower but gives a better quality juice. Once you have your lovely, sparkling machine(s), find a great place for them on your counter...you'll be using them a lot...so show them off!

Beyond the daily grind

Fresh ground herbs, spices and seeds...it's the ideal way to enjoy great flavor and zest with your meals, plus some wonderful health benefits to your diet. To create your own you'll need a blender, grinder or at least a mortar and pestle. If you have one, make sure it's in great working order. If you need to buy one, go with what works for you...there are several varieties to choose from to fit your style and budget. Grinding spice seeds helps to release the flavor for cooking; crushing the herbs helps to bring out the juices from the leaves.

A little sprout goes a long way

Sprouting...what is it and why should you do it? If you've never heard of sprouting...don't worry...a lot of folks haven't. Let me ask you a question...as a kid, did you ever do one of those science experiments where you grew mustard or water cress? That's basically sprouting...and we've all seen bean sprouts at a salad bar...even if we never tried them. Oh, and I'm sure you have a least one friend who has added a shot of wheat grass to a smoothie, right? So what's the point of it all and should you bother? Well, it's quite an easy thing to do that can really improve your health. How you ask? Great question...here's a quick list of the benefits of sprouting:

- Eating sprouts is easier on digestion because being young plants (once sprouted) the enzymes are available to help with digestion.
- They're more nutritious as they're picked/harvested at their prime giving the body a mass of vitamins, minerals, proteins, enzymes, and bio-flavanoids.
- It's economical...cheap to buy, cheap to grow...a few seeds go a long way!
- They're completely organic (providing one has purchased organic seeds).
- You can eat these at any time of the year...that means they're always *in-season*.
- Sprouts are totally fresh as they are grown and harvested quickly
- They're a versatile addition to your salads, soups, stir fry...whatever...and they add a new dimension to the look and taste of your foods.

If you've never sprouted before, check our Fact File G to get you started. It's really quite simple. You don't need much space or a green thumb to get the benefits of fresh sprouts! Now, what can you sprout? The list is truly endless, but here is a partial list to get you thinking: alfalfa, clover, fenugreek, broccoli and cabbage, radish, mustard, wheat grass, sunflower seeds, flax seeds, pumpkin, peas, quinoa (any grains actually), lentils and beans (mung, adzuki, chick pea, turtle and more).

Keeping Sharp

Sharp knives make life wonderful, so check out your entire set. If you can't remember the last time you sharpened your knives, then they're probably dull. If you don't have your own stone or sharpener, take them to an expert. There are several places that offer the service. And, don't forget what you'll be cutting, slicing and chopping on ...your chopping board. Is it clean...really clean? They often hold bacteria and contaminants so throw the awful, beaten up thing out. That's right just get a new one...they're cheap...buy two!

Out of the frying pan

Don't cook all of your fresh, natural food in old, chipped or pitted pots and pans. Cookware is made from a variety of materials, but you may not realize that most of these materials can leach into the food that you cook in them. Now, most of the time, this is harmless, but you should take care with some. For example, we used to think those non-stick surfaces were a great stride for healthy cooking (because less fat was needed to fry and sauté). However, as it ages, bits and pieces of this surface can flake off into our food...not such a good thing. Besides our non-stick 'friends', surfaces to be aware of are aluminum, anodized aluminum, copper, ceramic and plastics. The safest surfaces are probably stainless steel and iron, Bottom line, if you have old, tired cookware it may be time to restock your pots and pans. Again, here's a great excuse to go shopping for the right equipment if needed. Don't forget to look at our Details Diva Fact File F for the rundown on these surfaces and the six steps for safe cookware.

Dressing the part

You're going to be living a new life...make sure your dishes and tableware fit the part. Throw out all those old chipped plates, cups and glasses that are a breeding ground for bacteria if not meticulously washed and dried. You'll be much happier eating your tasty food and drinks from decent dishes and glassware! So, there you have it...another excuse to go shopping...and you get to brighten up your dining table.

Keeping it clean

Water is the one thing our bodies need more than anything else. You need to be sure you're getting the absolute purist water you can for drinking and cooking. It's not uncommon for people to have some sort of water filters...from filter pitchers to whole house filtration systems. But we don't always do a good job of keeping it operating at its best. So, if you have a filter system, be sure you change any replaceable parts...filters, cartridges, UV bulbs, etc. If you haven't yet taken the step...now is the time. You might even want to take the plunge as it were and buy yourself a distiller. Distilled water has even greater benefits...it not only supplies your body with needed pure water, but helps remove mineral deposits and other toxins from your body.

Less is more

There is actually one piece of equipment you could get rid of for good. That's your microwave! I know what you're thinking, "TRISHA! Are you nuts? I'm not getting rid of my microwave! I NEED it and mine is built in – I'd have a huge hole in my kitchen!!" I understand...it's like losing an arm or a leg. So, how about this...put a sticker on your microwave that says "DANGER! This piece of equipment can damage your food!!" That way you'll at least start thinking about what a microwave actually does while is cooks. What is that? Actually, it literally changes the molecular structure of the food...that doesn't sound too good, does it? Seriously, if it were such a healthy way to cook why would we call it "nuking" or "zapping" our food? And, it depletes the vitamins and minerals and makes many of the nutrients all but useless. So no matter how good the food you have is - cooking it in a microwave can undo all the good you're trying to do. So, if you do nothing else...please slap that sticker on your microwave!

Now that your kitchen is clean, your fridge and freezer are ready for stocking and your appliances are gleaming awaiting to serve you...it's time to talk about what you're going to be eating, when, how and why.

Step 3. MENU PLANNING

Prior planning ensures success

Okay, I know you're asking that age old question...what's for dinner? By now you're thinking, okay Trisha my cupboards are bare and I'm hungry...HELP! So, which foods do you choose and how do you plan a menu. Let's take it one step at a time...what should you be eating? Think back to the Hunter/Gatherer idea and living in Eden. Depending on the season, we need to have roots, leaves, fruits, seeds, nuts and blossoms. Percentage-wise it will look a bit like this:

o   25% vegetables

o   10 – 12% protein from lentils, beans, nuts, seeds

o   15% fruits and salads

o   35 - 55% whole grains

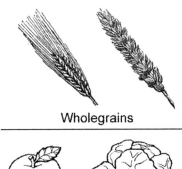

Wholegrains

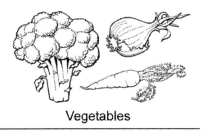

Vegetables

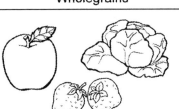

Fruits and Salads

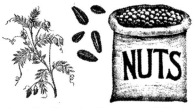

Lentils, Seeds, Beans and Nuts

Yes, I realize this does not add up to 100%. Don't worry, it is not new math...it's reality. You see, the exact percentages for you will depend on the season of the year, what's available locally, whether you are vegetarian, vegan or carnivore, if you have any diagnosed illness such as diabetes, where you live and if you're travelling, and of course...what you actually like!! I know, a novel concept, isn't it? This doesn't mean you can eat whatever you like, but I'm not going to insist carnivores give up meat, vegans eat eggs or that you have to somehow learn to stomach hot cereal if you detest it. 'Chapter 6: *The Good, the Bad & the Very Ugly*. Remember, this is a lifestyle change...so you have to be able to live with it.

You'll learn more about what types of foods to buy in the following step about shopping, but before we get into those details...it's time to talk menu planning.

When it comes to eating correctly, planning ahead is the key. It's when we don't know what we're going to have for our next meal that we tend to have problems staying on track. We don't have the right ingredients, not enough time to cook what we'd planned, or an imbalance in the types of food we're eating...too much of one group and not enough of the other. One other thing is color.... remember we eat with our eyes first, then smell and taste so ensure that your food choices look good on the plate. For specific sample menus, check out the 30-day plan at the end of this book.

Snacks

Snacks are an important part of a healthy diet. Women tend to go to the extreme and eat less and less to 'be healthy' when in fact; snacks – the right ones – keep your metabolism running all day long. That means you burn more calories and your body works more efficiently. It's vital to keep the metabolism working and the best way to do that is to provide regular fuel, or food. Snacks are not meals, but a little something to keep you going. Snacks can be the undoing of a healthy diet...especially in the workplace where well-meaning people bring in doughnuts, cookies and cake for everyone in the office. So, whether you work at home or in the office...be ready for that mid-morning or mid-afternoon moment when you need a quick bite. Ideal snacks are a handful of nuts or seeds, oatcakes with hummus, guacamole, crudités or some sliced fruit.

As you begin your menu planning, please look out the window. That's right...just do it. What season is it? You'll get the most nutrients and benefits from your food if you buy local, seasonal produce. So, when you hit the supermarket, just because they have cherries doesn't mean it's cherry season. Many fruits and vegetables are shipped in from other countries or hot house grown...so it may seem like you can choose anything you like, any time you want it. But, as you become aware of what's in season...you'll realize that what your body really craves is what's fresh not forced.

Step 4. SHOP 'TIL' YOU DROP
Getting the most out of your groceries

So, when you're at the store or market, how do you know if you're buying the right items? Well, with a little work, thinking seasonal and willingness to shop in different stores...or at least different aisles, you'll become a Healthy Tart shopper in no time. The majority of your diet is going to be made up of good carbohydrates. I know there's been a lot of confusion about carbohydrates lately, so I'd like to review what GOOD carbohydrates are...and yes good carbs are a vital part of your Healthy Tart diet. First, carbohydrates are not just breads and pastas...they include fresh fruits and vegetables. But, for a moment, let's talk about those 'grain products'. You need to only buy whole grains, with the hull intact. Why is that so important? Well to make white flour, white rice and most processed cereals...the whole grain is stripped of its out fiber. It makes the product easier to cook, but at the cost of vitamins, minerals, enzymes and fiber. They also process in the body faster creating extreme spikes in your blood sugar. Bottom line, refined carbohydrates are not good fuel for your body. You're left with a sugar or glucose crash and a craving for more. Remember this, any refined carbohydrate is processed by the body just like sugar...and we all KNOW we don't need more sugar in our diets. So, whole grain is the only grain! There's more information on good (and bad) carbohydrates in *Chapter Six: The Good, the Bad and the Very Ugly.*

Okay, with that in mind...how difficult can shopping be? Well, it can be rather tricky, depending on your habits. Many people were raised to bargain shop...clip coupons, buy in bulk and get what's on sale. Not a terrible trait, but think about the famous 'buy one get one free' idea. When was the last time you saw that offer attached to anything remotely healthy? While it may happen on occasion, never is the short answer to that. So, while healthy shopping doesn't have to be expensive, it will take some work and organization. Many of the major super market chains now feature excellent organic sections and provide lots of information about their healthy options. Visit their websites to see what they are offering. There are also new 'organic only' stores opening. These and your local shops are often great resources for recipes and cooking tips...so make friends with the local market owner and reap health and social benefits.

I've mentioned before about shopping for fruits and vegetables 'in-season'. This is another way those local shops can help...by confirming what's local and fresh as opposed to what's been shipped in from somewhere else. Shopping in season means only buy sprouts in winter when the first frost has hit them...peaches are a summer only fruit...and squash is a fall treat. The bottom line is that any food that is in season, in your country or area will make a great meal for you. Why? We are designed to eat this way as a way of cooling and heating our bodies according to the season. Plus, fresh and in-season always tastes better, so enjoy it!

While you want a supply of dried foods on hand...you don't want to buy in bulk unless you're feeding a large family and you have a quick turnover of food. You can always go shopping next week. If you have too much on hand, things will go stale (remember the mold I talked about?). And speaking of going stale...be careful not to buy stale food. Get your supply of lentils, nuts, seeds and such from a good supplier with a fast turnover. That way you know the foods have not been kicking around in the storeroom for years. Check for recent sell by dates on these items. And if you're not sure...ask for the sell buy date. If they don't have one...walk away and try somewhere else.

Liven things up with Herbs

Herbs are an important part of your new diet. They add loads of flavor, zest and health giving benefits to your meals. And, when trying to ease off salt, cut out junk food, and get back to the basics...the one thing people say they miss is flavor. Of course, what you're actually missing isn't so much the taste of food, but the flavor or too much salt, MSG and other food additives. That's why adding herbs (fresh or dried) can really make the difference for you. In fact, if you find yourself really craving salt, seaweeds are a great substitute. They have naturally occurring salt in their leaves and trust me; a strip of Kombu in a soup makes all the difference.

Now, the best way to get fresh herbs is to grow them yourself in a garden or even on a window ledge. But, if you just don't have a green thumb, visit the produce section for a variety of fresh herbs...the only limit is your willingness to try new flavors. Along with flavoring your food, many herbs offer therapeutic benefits as well. For a list of my favorites, check out Detail Divas Fact File H. You'll get some ideas for herbs to try and how they help your health!

There are a few other things to keep in mind as you wander the aisles for your fresh, natural bounty. If you can't find a good supply of oatcakes, you can make your own from a recipe in this book...they're easy! Select your protein from tofu, soya, beans, lentils, nuts and seeds. When getting stock for soups and gravies, reach for the low salt, yeast free items. Cooking and salad oils should be unrefined cold pressed virgin olive oil, sunflower, corn, sesame, walnut, peanut or safflower.

Dairy is often a big question for those wanting a healthy diet. And, in my opinion - based on experience - it depends on the state of health you're in, whether you have asthma or other respiratory problems, allergies, heart disease and so on, as to whether dairy is okay or an absolute no-no. Do think about this...the only being to drink milk after weaning is the human. Even cows do not carry on drinking their mother's milk, so why do we? Because of the calcium you say? Guess what...we can get that from other sources such as broccoli, kale, Swiss chard, almonds, as well as some from other food sources. Now if your health allows and you really must use cow's milk or dairy derivatives, please ensure they are of an organic source so they are free from hormones and antibiotics which are included in their feed and injected into the animals. However, please know there are also several dairy free options including rice milk, soy milk and oat milk and nut and seed butters that are options for your use.

And finally, while not ideal canned foods are a great standby. Keep in mind they are encased in metal, tin and possibly lead which may leach into the foods contained in the tin. For more information on metals, check out Chapter 6: *The Good, the Bad & the Very Ugly* and in the Detail Divas Fact File O.

Step 5. TART TIME MANAGEMENT
How to be a Healthy Tart on a busy schedule

WOW! How are you going to get it all done? I realize all of this shopping and chopping may at first feel like a chore, but in time life will get easier. You will have renewed energy and be able to handle your new lifestyle with ease. However, I've got six tips that will help make things easier right now. The key is preparation...from menus to shopping lists to actual food prep...plan ahead, know when you're going to do it and do as much in advance as possible. Most of your food can be prepared at least the day ahead, so work with your internal clock. If you're an early riser...prep your day's food each morning. If you're a night owl... prep your food the night before. If you're too tired to handle either one...that's a RED FLAG sign that your diet is so bad you're not resting well. But, if you follow my Ten Steps to Eden program, I promise this will all change for you in a matter of a few weeks. So, make the commitment now to do it for one month...the results will speak for themselves. Here are the Six Tips to Healthy Tart Time Management.

1. Shop once a week and keep a good supply of dry goods and cupboard ingredients. This ensures you always have fresh foods, but also a back up of those items you use more frequently...like whole grains.

2. Prepare all vegetables, salads, dressings in readiness for the following day, several days if the type of salad/vegetables you are preparing can be done that far ahead.

3. Keep a supply of mixed seeds and nuts in containers so that you can just throw them over your salads, fruits or whatever you are having them with.

4. Rice or other grains can be cooked up to three days in advance, but no more. If you do this, cook and cool immediately by dowsing with cold water. Don't leave it to cool on its own, as this can encourage bacteria to grow. If you're eating it right away...don't worry about it...this is for storing rice and grains only.

5. If growing your own sprouted nuts/seeds/beans ensure you rinse daily - at the same time as you wash and prepare vegetables.

6. Make your own fast food! Have homemade sauces ready to go...pre-wash vegetables...have quick-to-cook tofu or other main dishes in the fridge. You can have a healthy meal in less than 30 minutes...and that's as quick as running to the local fast food joint for a burger and fries...but oh so much better for you. Don't forget about snacks for the road. It's always good to have a bag of nuts or a piece of fruit with you for those times you get stuck away from home at mealtime.

Step 6. GOAL SETTING AND REWARDS
Doing it for yourself and celebrating your victories

There's a reason you're reading this book. Okay, maybe the title caught your eye...but it's more than that. You have something you'd like to change about yourself. Whether it's losing weight, getting fit, being less tired or just being happier with whom you are...you have a goal. This goal is just for you, not your husband, mother, kids or friends. And, that's the goal that matters...the one you do just for yourself. You deserve to reach that goal. So, think about it...what is it?

o   Lose ten pounds
o   Fit into that little black dress or those favorite jeans you've been dying to wear
o   Buy a whole NEW wardrobe
o   Surprise everyone at your school reunion
o   Participate in a marathon or other fitness challenge
o   Get off your high blood pressure medicine
o   Be able to play with your grandchildren
o   Get rid of the clothes in size 20, 18, 16, 14...and keep just one size forever!

So, how can you set good goals that raise the bar enough to challenge you, but don't overwhelm you into giving up altogether? Make your goals **S.M.A.R.T. goals.** That means your goals are:

Specific: Don't say, "I want to lose some weight." Instead say, "I want to lose 10 pounds in two months." Otherwise you won't know if you get there or where you're actually trying to go.

Measurable: How will you know when you achieved your goal? Is it marked on a calendar? Do you have weekly check-ins to see how you're doing? If your goal is to lose 10 pounds in two months, that means five pounds in one month and one and a quarter pound every week...you can measure that.

Attainable: Can you make this happen? Do you have the skills, resources, knowledge and desire to reach your goal? Can you get those needed things? If you want to lose weight, following the Healthy Tart plan helps make that *goal* attainable...I provide information, support and resources.

Realistic: This is really up to you...if you work at this, can it happen? An unrealistic goal (and unhealthy) would be "I'm going to lose 40 pounds in one month!" That's not very realistic and is likely to lead to discouragement and frustration...plus it's VERY unhealthy.

Timely: Having a timetable attached is the best way to
keep on track. Have weekly check-ins at the
same time, chart your progress. Just losing ten
pound is great, but if there's no timeframe
attached...there's no incentive to get started.
Maybe you have an event coming up...there's
your timeframe right there!

Remember that you can always increase or adjust your
goals...make new and different ones. It doesn't matter what it
is as long as it matters to you! And with every little goal you
reach, you need to celebrate...the right way. That does not
mean that when you lose five pounds you treat yourself to ice
cream. Food is fuel not reward, so you need to determine
things that will make you feel special and celebratory, but
not undo any of your great work. Any ideas? How about these:

- o   Get a manicure or pedicure
- o   Indulge in your favorite book
- o   Sneak off for an afternoon movie
- o   Sleep late on Saturday
- o   Get a massage or mud wrap
- o   Shop for antiques or shoes...anything you don't really
  need

Spend some time thinking about what feeds your soul, makes
you happy and brings you joy...little things count. Make a list
of these things and display them where you can see them.

That way you can think about them every day and KNOW these rewards will be yours...one with each goal you reach. So set the goals, but set the rewards too. Rewarding yourself will help keep you focused and on track and more committed to your own success. Keep a journal to track your goals and rewards. You can download one from my website.

Step 7. MOVE IT AND LOSE IT
Exercise, posture and movement

Almost everyone knows and understands the benefits of exercise. But, that doesn't mean you're doing it. Why? Lots of reasons, but the biggest one is probably you haven't found an exercise that suits you. If you hate working out with a group...you won't stick with an aerobics class. If you love organized sports...walking may bore you to tears. So, what is it that you enjoy doing? There are countless options out there including walking, stretching, dancing, pumping up the volume while vacuuming to your favorite music, belly dancing, pole dancing, yoga, Pilates, weight lifting, country line dancing...and so much more.

What about this scenario? Have you ever been excited about a new exercise program...gone all out and then just given up? That's not uncommon. You try to do too much, the intensity is too hard, you hurt and then you burn out. Still another challenge is that many people look at exercise as the last ditch effort to become slim and toned. They've been hoping that just cutting back on calories will be enough, but it isn't. Exercise increases circulation, improves oxygen flow through the vascular system, tones muscles, stimulates organs and systems of the body, increases strength and stamina, gives you control and power over your body and increases the release of endorphins (happy hormones).

You just cannot truly feel healthy unless you're out there moving, being flexible and being strong. That's why the important thing is for you to get out there and move your body... otherwise the body fluids become stagnant. You need to keep all that moving so that the blood carrying oxygen and nutrients can reach all the extremities of the body to regenerate the cells. This is called cell communication.

I realize you may have some challenges with exercise right now, but that's okay. Tune into your body and it will tell you what's going on inside and out. Start small and simple...make one little change each week. Before you know it you'll be hiking, biking, dancing, swimming...or whatever it is that you'd love to do.

Remember, exercise is a lifestyle change...just like your nutrition...so it's important that you do it the right way. That's why I've brought my good friend and colleague, Personal Trainer, Christin McDowell on board to help you get properly set up with a program tailored just for you. It's very important that you are careful and wise with how you go about your exercise program. That's why it's vital you visit the website and use Christin as your exercise counselor. She factors in your current lifestyle, exercise and medical history, your current physical measurements, body type, muscular imbalance assessment and your goals in creating your program. You just follow the necessary steps she gives you and you can rest assured you will see results, feel great and have the confidence you are getting some of the best training in the world. In fact, your program will fit you so well, you'll be motivated to stick with it because of the success you have. So, check out my website, www.TrishaStewart.com, go to the fitness section and you'll find out what you need to do to get started.

Step 8. DETOX OR NOT DETOX

The truth about detoxing your body

Sure, you've heard of detoxifications...maybe you've even tried one. But are they any good? What exactly do they do? Well, detoxing does just that...removes toxins from the body. How do we get toxins in our system? There are several reasons...some we control, some we don't. Excessive toxins in the system are caused by poor diet (too many fast foods, too much of the wrong types of fat, processed junk foods, soda, beer, wine and smoking), air pollution, heavy metals *[For more information on heavy metals and the damage they can do to your body, read Chapter 6: The Good, the Bad and the Very Ugly or check out the Detail Divas Fact File O]* including those amalgam fillings in your teeth, industrial toxins including deodorants, hair products and such, prescribed and over the counter medicines, even too many vitamin pills can cause a problem if the body is toxic.

So, what happens next? The liver will become congested, the kidneys will be overtaxed, you will probably be constipated, have diarrhea or a combination of both, your skin will be spotty due to the amount of toxins trying to get out through the skin, hair will be dull, nails will be brittle. If this sounds like you...then you might consider a detoxing.

Let me be clear right now... if you're very toxic there's really no point in doing a two-three day cleanse. This is just not long enough to help you. If fact a mini-cleanse will only serve to remove some fluids from the body, but would not allow enough time for the organs and systems to kick in. The liver may take quite a lot of clearing and stimulating. The 30-day plan I've created for you takes you through a gentle detox program. This will encourage you to lose weight, clean up the digestion, flush the kidneys and stimulate liver function. It's easy for beginners, but will also benefit those of you who have tried other detox or cleanse programs. The details for this detox is included in the 30-Day plan in Chapter 7: *Claiming your Healthy Tartness*. Down the road, you can look at doing other types of detox programs, with varying intensities and time-frames. My website, www.TrishaStewart.com has more details and steps for these. But, the 30-day plan is the best detox to start with and it's very doable for first timers.

Step 9. BODY TREATMENTS

Taking care of the outside package matters

I've talked a lot about the inside of the body...from digestion to elimination...from food intake to detox flushes. Now, it's time to talk about the outside of your body. To be truly healthy you need to also take care of your body's largest organ...the skin. It doesn't have to be complicated, but it does need to be consistent. The proper care of our skin helps us glow inside and out...improve our circulation and eliminates toxins.

To start... daily skin brushing is a great idea before you take your morning shower.

The skin is the largest excretory organ, covering your whole body, of course, and every day about 2 pounds of waste is eliminated through the pores, waste such as uric acid crystals, mucus and other body acids. Dry skin brushing literally sweeps away the dead skin and waste leaving a new skin...plus it's GREAT for the circulation!

Trisha, you may be asking...how do you brush your skin? It's very simple: Using a dry bristle, long handled brush or mitt (not nylon), start brushing up the body from the feet to the neck. Please use a softer brush for your face, but don't skip it. Also, DO NOT SCRUB your skin...it's too delicate for that.

And keep in mind that a little light brushing every day is far better than a "good thorough going over" once a week. As I've said, the idea is to brush away dead skin cells and excreted waste. If you can do this in the fresh air so much the better, but as your neighbors might not like it, you can certainly stand or sit on a towel in your bathroom.

Then there's your daily shower...it's also a form of natural therapy...hydrotherapy. Think about it. It's like a massage that stimulates your skin. It increases our circulation and cleanses the body of dead cells. Plus, all the tiny hair follicles on your skin are stimulated, allowing body fluids to move out.

And here's something surprising...if you were living and eating as you should...you wouldn't need deodorant. I'm serious! Perspiration is nothing more than our fluids moving out of our body. You need to secrete sweat in order to stay healthy. But what do people do?? Apply a chemical loaded deodorant, anti-perspirant to block the hair follicles and cover up the body odor. Well, if the body was clean inside because it was fed with good natural foods and lots of clean spring water, only sweet smelling fluids would come through onto the skin. Makes you wonder doesn't it? Now, I'm not telling you to stop using deodorant, but please buy a natural deodorant without all the chemicals. Plus, you might find you need it less once you get on track and get back to Eden...and your skin will thank you!

Finally, there is necessary relaxation. Your body needs to rest, to recoup, and one of the best ways is to take a bath in lovely warm water with perhaps some herbs or flowers floating in the water. For relieving muscle aches and relieving stress you can try an Epsom bath...but please NOT if you have high blood pressure or a heart or kidney condition. So, depending on your needs you could keep it relaxing, make it stimulating or even soothing for sore muscles...all depending on what you drop in the water. Another thing to keep in mind is that alternating hot and cold water will stimulate and tone your skin. It's a little shocking to the system at first, but your body will come to crave the alternating feelings and you'll feel amazing.

So, whether your shower or bathe...water is an important part of your skin care. And great skin...from the inside out...is a major part of being a Healthy Tart.

Step 10. BRINGING IT ALL TOGETHER
Cooking & Juicing for the Healthy Tart

So, you've got all the bits and pieces to this puzzle and it's time to put them together. This last step is some of the how-to in putting all the previous steps into play. In other words, you've cleaned and restocked your kitchen with the right foods and equipment; you've planned your menus, set goals, and now you're ready to GO.

The Juice of Life

Let's get started with juicing. I mentioned getting a good juicer in Step Two, and it's important that you do not use a blender or smoothie maker as they don't produce the juice. However they are great for making smoothies! Okay, let me share some of the benefits of juicing. I know it can be difficult to chew your way through lots of fruit and vegetables, especially if you are in a hurry. So, juicing together a mixture of fruits and vegetables into one glass provides you a great tasting way to get some vitamins, minerals and enzymes packed in FAST.

Now keep in mind that you do lose some of the wonderful pulp when you juice...and that's a loss of great fiber which helps clean or 'scour' the colon. And, because you're not chewing, which exercises the facial muscles, you're not producing as many of the enzymes to break down the fruit and vegetables. Still, I believe that the combination of juicing, eating raw foods and enjoying cooked foods is the perfect way to health and happiness.

Now, here are some of the basic steps to juicing:

- First of all set up your juicer, if possible near a sink so that you can immediately put the used components into hot water to rinse off.
- Keep the chopping boards and knives nearby, almost set up your own juice bar.
- Purchase only fresh - if possible organic - ingredients (throw out the moldy, old, wrinkled stuff)
- Buy whatever produce is in season as these will have been naturally ripened
- A good selection of leafy greens such as kale, cabbage, spinach, watercress, rocket, parsley, lemon grass, plus broccoli, courgette, cucumber, beetroot, celery, carrots, sprouted beans and legumes, apples, avocado, pineapple, banana, melon, lemons and limes (wax free) ginger root, sprouted alfalfa or any other sprouts. Check some of the recipes I've included in chapter seven!
- Do not always choose fruit or sweet options. Carrots, apples, etc. provide amazing sweetness when added to greens and other ingredients, which will give you hours

of energy. But fruit alone, while it offers great energy, will not sustain you as well.

- You can add coconut milk, soy milk or yogurt or nut milks but remember these will be more of a smoothie and not to be encouraged on the two day juicing.
- Wash all produce...even organic as people during picking and packing will have been handling those products.
- You may need to peel some fruits, such as pineapple. Some juicers can handle tough rinds and peels, but personally I don't think you can clean the outside of a pineapple that well! But, make your own decisions...nothing you do will be wrong...experiment and have fun!
- You may need to cut pieces to fit your juicer. Don't ever force large chunks as it will only ruin your machine.
- It is best to prepare the juice that you are going to drink immediately, you can keep some in a flask or the fridge but it will not be of the same quality or contain as many vitamins, minerals or enzymes as freshly prepared.
- Try to utilize the pulp rather than waste it. Put it into a soup or casserole dish, or if all else fails...feed it to your dog!

Again...have fun!! I have included some recipes in Chapter Seven, but feel free to make up your own. As you learn what you like, don't forget variety to give yourself a wide range of nutrients.

Let's get cooking!!
Some of you may already be taking steps to prepare and cook your foods in healthier ways. But, for some of you out there some basics may need a new twist. I've talked a lot about using only the freshest ingredients possible...but it's also important to cook things as close to when they'll be eaten as possible. Bearing in mind any time management tips you're using to make life a bit easier, of course.

So, you've got fresh foods, everything is ready to go and now what? Well, if you're sautéing some veggies and tofu...try stir frying in a bit of vegetable stock instead of butter or oil. You can still drizzle and toss in a bit of olive oil (for example) towards the end of cooking, so you get great flavor and reduce the amount of calories. Look for ways to bake, roast and broil foods that don't require adding anything but fresh spices and herbs. And, for those that were raised on 'boiled to hell' vegetables...if you can't take them raw...steam them so they cook quickly and still maintain their nutrients.

Remember your one percent changes here and make steps in improving the methods and approaches you use to cook your meals. Be willing to try something new, experiment and have some fun. And, I've gone through almost every grain, vegetable and fruit offering ways to prepare...so check out Detail Diva Fact File I for the Food Prep & Cooking for Healthy Tarts.

Mark your calendar

That's right...you've got all the steps you need and it's time to pick your start date. I've created an easy-to-follow 30-day plan that sets you on the path straight to Eden. Within 4-weeks you'll be feeling happier, healthier and more alive than ever before. Of course, there may be a few bumps along the way. I mean after all you're changing your lifestyle, not just your outfit. So, check out Chapter 5: *Obstacles to Eden* and remember...if you have challenges with following the 30-day plan you can contact the Trisha Stewart Team and we'll help customize a plan specific to your health needs and challenges.

Chapter 5

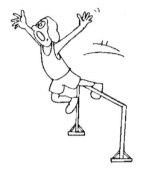

Obstacles to Eden

The saying goes... "The road to hell is paved with good intentions"...but do they really get you to where you want to go? They certainly get you started and we all MEAN to do the things we say we're going to do...well, most of us...at least when it comes to our health. You really do intend to hit the gym, cut out the sugar, and eat more vegetables...right? So what happens? You start out with all the enthusiasm of a small child at Christmas...then a few weeks into it you lose steam...it gets more difficult and before you know it you've given up all together. But, you feel you've got good reasons, don't you? In the years I've been seeing patients, trust me I've heard them all. time, money, family, work commitments,...bad knees, bad back, bad timing...can't do it alone...can't do it with that person...guess what they all have in common...they're excuses. Some seem legitimate...there are only 24 hours in a day, some seem insurmountable...a bad back can prevent you from certain exercises. But, all excuses are equal...so let's get down to what's really going on.

Life is hard...it's challenging and there are obstacles that get in the way of reaching our health goals...any goals for that matter. But Oprah Winfrey has a great way to look at challenges. She says, "Challenges are gifts that force us to search for a new center of gravity. Don't fight them. Just find a different way to stand." So, I ask you...how bad do you want it? That's what it comes down to. If you want something badly enough, you'll work for it, work through the obstacles and – as Oprah says – find a different way to stand. Okay, Trisha...that sounds great in theory...but how? What do I do when I feel weak, want to give up, have temptation hit me right in the face? Well, let's take a look at some of the most common obstacles.

Obstacle. If I start this program, I'll end up cooking multiple meals every day...mine, my husband's, my kid's...it's just going to be too difficult.

Solution. The answer to not having to cook multiple meals...don't do it! There are ways for you to make meals that are healthy for you and palatable to your kids and/or spouse. Plus as you start to eat a bit healthier, your family will get used to the idea and actually enjoy the nutritious, healthy meals you create...especially when they see the results you'll be getting.

Obstacle. My husband loves meat and potatoes and we like to eat together...even if it's really late when he gets home.

Solution. First, don't try to change everything in everyone's diet right away. For some of you, you'll be making some really big changes...so taking it one step at a time actually works out better in the long run. Remember this is NOT a diet, but a lifestyle change. So, don't feel you have to swipe the steak off the table on day one, but be sure you're adding lovely organic vegetables and healthy grains. Then, as you contemplate your choices...you focus on the healthy alternatives...eating less and less of what you're eliminating from your diet. As far as eating late goes...do it as little as possible. It's not good for anyone to eat too late at night (refer back to Chapter Three "It's what's on the inside that counts" for more details on digestion) but sometimes it happens. If you know you're hubby is getting home late, go ahead and eat at the correct time, then just sit with him while he eats. It's really just your company he wants. Now, if he really does want to you dine with him, keep your plate small and simple...a few more veggies, a bit of salad or grain...you get the idea. If you stick to your guns and plan ahead, you'll be better equipped to stay on track...and thereby get better results. And, what's one of the biggest results you're likely to get? Your spouse is going to see your increased energy, improved health and happier life and begin to want these changes for himself. And you can help him do just that. Don't forget to get him a copy of "You don't have to be Superman to be a Healthy Stud Muffin." I've taken the core of Healthy Tart and adapted it for the men in our lives and their unique health and nutrition concerns (check the website for the release date).

Obstacle. I have kids! They love their pizza, burgers and fast food. In fact, more often than not, it is all they'll eat.

Solution. Okay, I'm not going to tell you how to parent (that's an entirely different book by some other expert), but I have to ask...who is the parent? How are your kids getting this fast food? Who's picking up the pizza on the way home from work? Ouch! I know it hurts, but it's often true. So...next question. Why are you reading this book? Do you want to be healthier? Feel healthier? Do you want to keep your children from experiencing some of the same challenges and frustrations, perhaps even health risks that you're facing? Okay, so do them a favor...change their lifestyle before they get to feeling like you do. Sure, kids will likely do what they like when hanging out with their friends but you can work to improve their health while they're with you. By the way...I know dealing with kids and their diets can be an entire topic on its own. That's why I'm writing "You don't have to be a Health Nut to be a Healthy Pumpkin." This book addresses the special dietary and health concerns for children twelve and under.

Obstacle. Ok, but how do I actually stop a kid from eating too much junk food?

Solution. Simply, you make it less available. Make fast food an occasional (no more than once a week) treat...not the norm. As I said, they're likely to sneak a few chips or chocolate or whatever with their friends, but control what's in your kitchen. However, please take caution and don't try to change everything overnight. If you make too many changes at once you'll get rebels and there's no need for that. Start slowly by offering healthier snack alternatives and they'll adapt.

Obstacle. What do I do during the holidays or at birthday parties and other celebrations? There's always so much temptation around.

Solution. It is hard to say no to your favorite holiday treat or just one piece of your niece's birthday cake. But, remember this...there will always be an event, gathering or celebration around the corner. So, if you always make an exception for every event...that becomes your normal behavior...not the healthy living choices. That means at some point you just have to make some tough decisions. Remember what I asked you earlier in the chapter? How bad do you want it? That may seem simple, but it helps when you're looking face to face with temptation. It makes you ask the bigger question...what's more important: your health or a piece of cake? Don't panic!! That doesn't mean you can never have indulgences...it means you are in control of your actions and they're your decisions. As you become healthier, have more energy and are just living a better quality of life...most if not all of those 'celebration/holiday' temptations lose their power.

Obstacle. I dine out a lot and I find it's almost impossible to eat well in most restaurants. How do I stick with my plan then?

Solution. Whether it's dinner in a restaurant or dinner at a best friend's...limited menus can be a real challenge. However, most dining events are booked in advance, so that gives you time to plan ahead. It's okay to alert your host to your dietary situation as long as you're pleasant about it. Don't demand to be catered to but you can easily say something like, "I'd love to come to your home for dinner...it will be wonderful to see you. Oh, and I should let you know I'm choosing vegetarian options these days." With enough notice hosts are usually happy to keep you food options in mind while they select the menu. Another option is to offer to bring along a dish you can enjoy, again wording is important. Try something like, "Oh, it will be fun to catch up and, since I'm eating a particular diet these days, how about if I bring a dish along that fits my diet. I'll bring enough for everyone to try and you won't have to worry about altering your menu for the night."

With restaurants you've got even more flexibility. If you aren't familiar with their menu, check it out to get the details (give them a call, look them up online...). If you know you're going somewhere one evening you can eat a heartier lunch and keep it simple for dinner. Surprise outings? Stick with vegetables and salads and skip the bread. And for those die-hard carnivores, select fish or plainly cooked meat...unless it's during the 30-day plan, then you must adhere to the vegetarian options. Don't assume the vegetarian options are healthy...many are loaded with cheese and simple carbohydrates. And, don't be afraid to ask for no sauces, substitute potatoes for extra vegetables or grilled instead of fried. Best to skip dessert...even fruit after a meal is not useful because it causes the other foods to go too quickly through the digestive process leaving you feeling hungry again.. A fruit starter would be better. In fact it's okay to order from a menu the wrong way around, the restaurant is there to serve you food in any way you wish.

Obstacle. I'm really busy with work, meetings and family obligations...I don't have the time it takes to cook everything from scratch.

Solution. Everyone is busy...we all have just a bit too much to do every day, whether we put that on ourselves or it's heaped on by others...it's difficult. The key to not feeling overwhelmed is planning...from menus to shopping to time management. Believe it or not, with the right prep...you can have a home-cooked real meal ready in 30-minutes. I feel these things are so important that they are all part of the 10-step program to Eden. So, for further details on working with a busy schedule, check out the 10-Steps again and focus on steps three, four and five.

Obstacle. My friend always seems to sabotage my diet and exercise efforts. How do I handle this?

Solution. It's a hard fact to accept, but we all have or have had someone in our life who struggles to be happy for us and support our successes. Please understand that it's usually not a conscious effort. They just see your success mirroring their own failure and rather than change themselves, they try to change the image back to something less threatening. This sabotage can take the obvious form of plying you with your favorite 'no-nos' or it can be as subtle as questioning the validity of the program you're using. This can easily derail you, but here are some tips:

You're doing this only for yourself...so your choices are about you not them. And ask yourself, "How bad do you want it?"

Include them in the program. If you get them started on the same program you will become great allies. And, even if they opt out...they'll have a better idea of why you're doing what you're doing.

1. Plan ahead for your own version of healthy indulgences so you can fall back on those snacks when something fat-laden and sugar loaded is passed your way.
2. Stay away. If you have a friend who truly just doesn't want you to improve yourself and feel healthier, you may need to distance yourself from them or at least limit the amount of time you're spending together until you are solid in your new lifestyle.

Obstacle. I'm on a really tight budget and buying all that expensive organic foods is just not realistic for me.

Solution. Shopping and eating healthy is no more expensive that eating lots of processed products...especially if you shop smart. Sometimes good for you foods DO go on sale and some things, like rice and grains, can be purchased in bulk as long as you're eating it consistently. Also don't forget to review your entire budget to see where your money is really going. A few fast food meals can equal a week's worth of fresh lunches and dinners. If you're eating the right foods, you can eliminate many of the supplements you've been purchasing (although never go off any medication without your doctor's approval). Plus, as you get healthier, you lose less time from work and have more energy to have fun...so you're paying yourself with more time and better energy. Bottom line...think "big picture"...look for sales...buy in bulk when appropriate.

Chapter 6

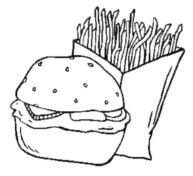

The Good, the Bad and the Very Ugly

You've read a lot about my views on what to put into your body, when and why...from fruits to veggies to detox solutions to supplements. But, I know some of you are out there wondering about some of the things I have NOT mentioned or written about in this book...so far. So, that's what this chapter is all about...a few facts on how to get the most 'good' from the right foods, and – of course - those things you should eliminate from your diet (or at least cut back on drastically). More importantly, you're going to learn the reasons, or the 'whys', behind my choices. I say choices because even though I feel VERY strongly about what are the best foods to eat...it's still a choice. It is my choice (although at this point in my life I can see no other way for myself) and it's about your choice. In other words, I'm not going to tell you that if you don't eat exactly the way I do you are wrong or a bad person. However, I am going to share with you the culmination of my years of research, experience and expertise so you will understand why I have made the food decisions I have. Then, it will be up to you to make your own decisions...but at least you'll have the truth. Fair enough?

THE GOOD

My entire book is filled with "the good stuff" of fresh fruits, vegetables, nuts, grains and seeds. And, I believe in eating organically whenever possible to ensure you're getting the most benefit from your food without the worry of added hormones or pesticides. For a detailed list of suggested good foods, review the 10-steps and check out the shopping list in Chapter Seven: *Claiming your Healthy Tartness.*

Now, here is where I have to say I am not a big fan of taking supplements. There are cases when I would advise the use of them, if there are major deficiencies due to illness, disease, if you're are working and stretched to the limit there are certain supplements I would advise, if you are a sportsperson and utilizing every nutrient and more. The problem is there is little regulation on the quality and quantity of vitamins and minerals out there. Remember, it is not just what you eat, it is what you absorb. So, if your digestive system is working to its full potential and you are actually absorbing nutrients from an excellent diet, then there shouldn't be a need to supplement. But, if that's not the case then it's great you're reading this book as your health will certainly improve; as indeed will your absorption. We will, of course, be happy to recommend some top quality supplements should they be required.

Unless you are on recommended supplements, I believe that your budget would be put to better use by buying more organic foods that give you the nutrients you need. That's the real Back to Eden lifestyle I believe in for everyone. I'm sure you're thinking, 'but Trisha...there are some minerals we can't get from foods'...or 'I have allergies that keep me from eating certain foods'. I know I know...but there are more sources for most vitamins and minerals than you probably realize. So if the 'traditional' food source is not available, causes allergic reaction (oh – that's a completely different book...believe me), try an alternative source. Now, I don't expect you to know what those other sources might be...so I've created a nutrient chart (Fact File J) to explain what vitamins and minerals actually do for your body and what foods have those nutrients. As you're beginning this program, you might want to have this list along with your shopping list. That way if you see you're really missing out on certain nutrients, you can quickly refer to the list to complete your shopping list.

THE GOOD & THE BAD

When we break our food down into its most basic form...proteins, carbohydrates and fats...there is good and bad in all of it. We need all three pieces of the nutrition puzzle to become a real picture of health...to become the picture of a Healthy Tart. It's the source and amount of these three building blocks that can often cause us problems and health challenges. So, let's take a look at the good & bad of proteins, carbs and fats.

Proteins

Proteins play a vital role in the growth and repair of your body cells and tissues. They are also involved in the synthesis of enzymes, plasma (blood) proteins, antibodies (immune) and some hormones, and provide energy...although only after any handy carbohydrates are burned.

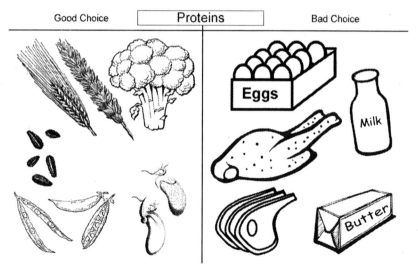

So, what are the best sources for protein? I believe they include whole grains, beans, legumes and some vegetables. These are also classed as slow release or complex carbohydrates, so it is not hard to get all your protein, carbs and fiber in one meal. Believe it or not we do NOT need to eat meat, poultry, dairy, eggs or fish to get good quality protein.

"But, Trisha, give up meat", you carnivores are asking!! Well, remember what I said about it being your choice? I've made a choice based on the good sources of protein available in vegetarian foods. And, here are the reasons I do not promote the use of animal proteins (based on several studies):

- Higher incidence of colorectal cancer
- Constipation leading to diverticulitis
- Higher incidences of colitis or other inflammatory digestive problem
- Headaches, bad breath
- Raised acidity leading to gall stones, liver damage, kidney stones and renal damage, bone loss/osteoporosis as the body excretes more calcium to maintain mineral balance
- Raised cholesterol
- Higher risk of heart disease
- Higher risk of diabetes or diabetic related symptoms
- Higher risk of obesity in adults and children
- Growth hormones and antibiotics used in mass producing cattle, sheep, pigs and poultry possibly causing infertility and who needs antibiotics!

For me, the benefits and increased vitality of a vegetarian lifestyle far exceed the risks of eating meat. I've provided a more detailed look at my viewpoint in Fact File J. And, I believe, after you've completed the 30-day plan...you will truly crave less meat and be feeling better. So, stick with it and even if you can't cut out meat completely, do make the commitment to yourself to cut back...eat less fatty cuts and focus on organic meats...and increase your other sources of protein. Your body will thank you!

Carbohydrates

Carbohydrates...they've been given a bad rap lately, but they are still the best source of energy out there. Because carbohydrates are easy to digest and a quick source of concentrated energy, athletes often "carbo-load" before big games, races or events for sustained energy. And, along with providing rapid energy and heat, they 'spare' proteins (leaving them to repair and build tissue). However, the wrong type of carbs and any carbs eaten in excess are stored as fat deposits under the skin (not great if you are trying to lose weight!). Remember, I said there is good and bad to everything. It's that bad side...excess stored as fat and simple carbohydrates (I'll get to them in a minute) that have given ALL carbs a bad name. And, that is what's caused the influx of "No-Carb" and "Lo-Carb" diets that in the long run are not healthy or maintainable.

Good Choice | Carbohydrates | Bad Choice

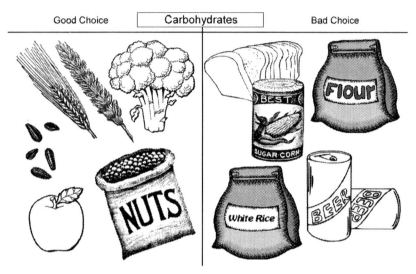

But, it's really very simple...it's the quality of the carbohydrate that makes all the difference...it's about whether they are simple or complex carbohydrates. Let me explain the way the carbs work simply:

- Refined or simple carbs and sugars cause your blood sugar to rise rapidly, and unless you are regularly exercising there will be too much glucose in the blood stream so the body will dump it as fat deposits. Your blood sugar levels then crash, and you will experience lethargy, poor concentration, palpitations and/or a feeling of anxiety and even sweating. You will crave more food, coffee and other stimulants. You can see the vicious cycle. Believe it or not, years ago, even top athletes thought eating sweets (nothing but simple sugar) would give them a boost. Now we know that even though athletes don't dump excess sugars like sedentary folks, this was not and still is not a good way to get energy. The problem is that a lot of office bound workers are eating simple carbs (or sugars) as if they were built, trained and exercised like athletes. But, they're sitting around all day, which means massive dumping of sugar or glucose as it will be by then, into those fat deposits.

- On the other hand, the slow release carbs from the starchy vegetables, grains and beans help to balance out the blood sugar levels. They release the sugars or glucose into the blood stream slowly...providing long-lasting, even energy. That's why porridge in the morning is far more sustaining than crunchy nut cornflakes!

Here's a quick list of sources for complex carbohydrates:

- Root vegetables like pumpkin, squash, carrot, beetroot, sweet potato, white potato and corn.

- Low glycaemic vegetables (that have little impact on blood sugar) including asparagus, aubergine, broccoli, brussel sprouts, cabbage, cauliflower, celery, courgette, cucumber, endive, fennel, garlic, kale, lettuce, mange tout, mushrooms, onions, peas, peppers, radish, rocket, runner beans, spinach, spring onions, tomatoes (technically a fruit), watercress and so on.

- Whole grains, rice, quinoa, buckwheat, millet, cornmeal, couscous, whole rye, whole wheat.
- Legumes, lentils, peas, chick peas, split peas.
- Beans: soy, pinto, borlotti, butter, kidney, flageolet, haricot and black eyed peas
- Nuts and seeds

And, for the VERY UGLY – here's a list of those simple carbohydrates that you need to avoid. I know they might taste good, but please think about what they're doing to your body…and how they are NOT delivering good nutrition.

- Simple starches including white bread, pasta (yes, it's just flour, water and sometimes a bit of egg), white rice, dinner rolls, buns, sweetened cereals and crackers
- Sweets: cookies, cakes, chocolates, soda pop, candy
- Frozen pizzas, microwave dinners, potato chips, roasted and salted nuts
- Sweetened fruit: canned fruits, jams, jellies and juices. (I know…juice is from fruit, but it's so loaded with fructose, natural sugar that's okay in one piece of fruit, but too concentrated in juice).

The information on carbohydrates can be confusing, I know! You need to be wary of foods that provide what we call empty calories as they lead to weight gain and feeling sluggish and tired. For a great reference of foods and how they affect your blood sugar level. See Glycaemic Index in Fact File L.

FATS

It is very clear that over the last 10 years people have been eating too much fat and oil. Not only is it naturally occurring in the food we eat, but in so many of the packaged and prepared foods you buy. And, while some food companies and restaurants are taking steps to change that...it's really up to you to cut back. Of course, the logical step is to avoid fatty foods wherever and whenever possible...sounds good, right? But there are some oils and fats which we need in our diets to keep us healthy...so like good and bad proteins and carbohydrates...there are good and bad fats.

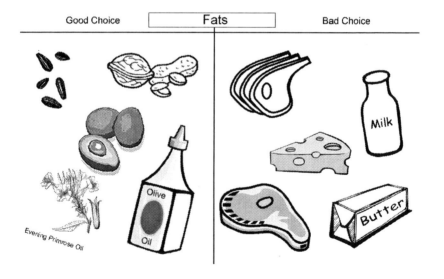

The idea to "cut out the fat" led to the extreme low fat diet craze. And that is leading to problems such as depression,

PMS and menopausal symptoms. In fact, too little fat in the diet has been connected to more cases of depression, mental illness and it would appear that more children have ADHD...there even seems to be an increase in people with Schizophrenia. The problem is that people just cut something out of their diet without knowing the risks and how to replace what they are missing with another source. So, let's look at what fats you DO need in your diet and how to eliminate or cut back on what you don't.

There are two basic types of fatty substances which come from food: fats and cholesterol. Believe it or not, we need cholesterol to help make bile to emulsify fat, sex hormones and protect the sheath around the nerves. But, there's no need to take in any sources of cholesterol, your liver makes plenty to cover our required 2,000 mgs per day.

So, what about fats? Fat becomes an energy source when we have no carbohydrates stored and as padding to keep internal organs from bouncing around. Fats are also needed as protection around the nerves and to help keep cell membranes fluid so cells can change shape as needed, for instance, when red blood cells need to squeeze through capillaries.

The problem is that we consume two types of fat...*saturated* and *unsaturated*. We need to avoid saturated fats that increase our blood cholesterol and body fat. Saturated fat includes butter, lard, bacon grease, margarine and solid (hydrogenated) vegetable shortening. On the other hand, *unsaturated* contain the essential fatty acids (or EFAs)...that's the type of fat your body needs. The best sources for EFAs are nut and seed oils, fish oils and vegetable oils

So what do these good fats...these EFAs...do for you? Fatty acids can be converted in the cells of our bodies into substances called prostaglandins. These cellular messengers affect blood clotting, blood vessels, tissue response to hormones and transmission of nerve impulses and more. The fats from shellfish, dairy and red meat tend to become those prostaglandins which increase inflammation in the body and encourage blood clotting. Those from vegetable, nut and seed oils tend to do the opposite. In fact, aspirin works by blocking the conversion of fatty acids into inflammatory prostaglandins. This is why it helps reduce the risk for heart disease and certain cancers.

Some seed and fish oils are more powerful in reducing inflammation and clotting than others. Cold or deep ocean fish contain more of the 'omega-3' fatty acids which reduce blood clotting and reduce the risk for heart disease. They are also particularly good at reducing joint inflammations like bursitis and the common form of arthritis called 'degenerative joint disease'. However, fish oils may be laden with mercury;

which is why I recommend seed oils. And, borage seed oil contains a high amount of 'omega-6' fatty acids good for reducing inflammation in the skin (eczema), and lungs (asthma), and this oil has been particularly effective in reducing pain and inflammation from autoimmune diseases such as rheumatoid arthritis and lupus. *By the way...I have had some successes with Borage seed oil in conjunction with dietary changes and supplements to treat patients with all sorts of hormonal issues, including stress, PMS and Menopause.*

There is one type of oil which contains a significant amount of all the essential fatty acids (omega-3, -6 and -9) is flax oil. Be aware, however, that because flax is so highly unsaturated, its fatty acids can become oxidized easily. Oxidation causes free radical formation which can cause inflammation and impaired immune function, counteracting any benefits from taking this oil.

So how do you modify your diet to help reduce your risk of heart disease while still getting these essential fatty acids? First, avoid all saturated fats and fried foods whenever possible. And, if you must butter your bread, use real butter rather than an artificially saturated fat like margarine which may be hydrogenated. Just remember to use as little as possible and try substituting olive oil instead. Keep total fats down to 20% of calories. On a 1500 calorie diet, 300 calories from fat (or 2 1/2 Tbsp oil) per day, preferably a seed oil or seeds and nuts. Consume omega-3 & 6 fats through flax and other seeds and nuts, and if like, you can eat cold water fish including halibut, cod, salmon or tuna up to twice a week (watch out for mercury in fish). If you have a specific health problem, try using an essential fatty acid supplement such as those mentioned above, plus an antioxidant nutrient.

THE VERY UGLY

There are a few things I want to touch on that are the ugly side of nutrition...sugars, alcohol, cheese, heavy metals and molds. I already addressed the 'very ugly' side of eating meat in the section on proteins...so re-read that if you need more incentive! I believe the more information you have; the easier it will be for you to make wise choices for your health.

SUGAR

Refined sugar is that white (or even brown colored) crystallized product that people spoon into their drinks, poor over cereal and add to cakes, cookies and more. But, the even bigger problem is the massive amount added to junk food and so called "healthy" products labeled as "low fat" or "fat free". Called everything from sugar to high fructose corn syrup (Complete sugar list: Fact File M), these simple sugars cause a swift change in blood sugar levels due to the rate the body converts them to glucose. This quick rise in blood sugar and energy is followed by a swift crash...leaving you wanting (and feeling like you need) even more sugar.

This endless cycle leads to an excess of sugar, which WILL sit as fat deposits...so yes, sugar does make you fat...not just fat loaded foods. In fact, high sugar diets are a leading cause of obesity, diabetes and heart disease. And, Candida actually thrives on sugar...so if you struggle with these bacteria...natural sugars are a real problem. Even fructose, which occurs naturally in fruits, will build up the amount of actual sugars/glucose/glycaemic load that is passing through your body.

What's even more frustrating is that artificial sweeteners affect blood sugar levels just like natural sugars. And even products like Stevia or Agave-nectar, which have less impact on the blood sugar, still feed your 'sweet tooth' and do little to alleviate your addiction. So, clearly the less sugar of any sort you have in your diet, the healthier you're going to be. Attention Detail Divas: If you have sugar cravings and need more information on natural and artificial sweeteners, please check out Fact File M.

ALCOHOL

Around the world (or most of it) it seems we're drinking more...at least more wine. And a big reason for that is that we keep hearing wine is good for us. Red wine is full of bioflavanoids...just like the berries we love to eat. Plus, wine is fruit (grapes), so what can be wrong with that? Well, in moderation quality wine can be beneficial according to scientists. Moderation, by the way, is just a glass or two at most.

So, what is quality wine and what should you be looking for when buying a bottle or glass of wine? Ideally, you should drink organic wine...made from organic grapes, grown in organic soil with no spraying of synthetic fungicide, fertilizer and herbicides. But, many people, maybe you're one of them, are sensitive to Sulphur Dioxide (sulfites) that occur naturally on the grape. The real problem is that sulfites are also added to wine to preserve and help to kill off bacteria. So, while no wine can be completely sulfite-free, you can search for wine without ADDED sulphites

For those who are interested, you can go one step nearer to Eden and buy biodynamic grown wines. Biodynamic is the teaching of Rudolf Steiner that uses homeopathic sprays and herbal preparations with estate-made composts to increase soil fertility and strengthen and protect the vines from pests and disease. Believe it or not, lunar cycles, earth rhythms and astrology are also employed to ensure that activities in the vineyard are correctly timed. But, no matter how much love, care and natural processes have gone into growing the grapes; once they're harvested it's often another story. So, for my wine drinkers out there...just read labels, do your research, buy organic and ALWAYS drink in moderation!

Now, let's look at beer. Most often made from hops (a natural plant from the nettle and cannabis family) or from malted barley and some other grains you can search for beer from organic plants. That's a start at any rate. In fermenting beer, yeast, water and other ingredients are added to create every brands unique variety. The other ingredients may or may not be organic...so check where they are grown and brewed for authenticity.

There are many types of alcoholic beverages, far too many to mention, but what I want to tell you is that the derivative from each and every one of them whether made from fruit, grain or whatever, is alcohol. And too much of it can be a bad thing. Here's a quick list of what can befall you if you drink too much:

- Acidity, peptic ulcers, gastritis, pancreatitis
- Inability of the small intestine to absorb nutrients due to damage which may cause a shortage of Vitamin B1 (thiamine) which is required for normal brain, heart, nerve and muscle action
- High blood pressure, heart muscle disease and heart failure
- Disturbed sleep

- Gout due to the build of uric acid
- Kidney and liver disease
- Higher risk of mouth, tongue and esophagus cancer
- Birth defects, miscarriages, premature babies etc if Mothers drink alcohol whilst pregnant
- Fertility problems
- Increased risk of diabetes
- Impaired judgment
- Anxiety
- Depression
- Confusion

So, as I have said...and backed by science...there are some health benefits to a nip or two, but drinking TOO much can have a serious affect on your health.

CHEESE

Don't panic! I am not going to say do not eat cheese!! People have been eating it for years, and it can be a source of protein and some vitamins. However, it's important that you know cheese is linked to respiratory problems, migraine headaches, excess mucus and sinus problems, snoring and allergies/intolerances. So, I wanted you to have a bit more information so you can make your own decision from a place of knowledge.

Cheese is a dairy food, typically made from the milk of a cow, goat or sheep. It is made by coagulating or thickening milk to create curds, which are then separated from the liquid (or whey). It's then processed and matured to produce a wide variety of cheeses. Sounds okay, right? Well, milk is coagulated by the addition of rennet (an enzyme) and the usual source of rennet is the stomach of slaughtered newly-born calves. Wow, that's not very tasteful...is it? Now, in vegetarian cheese making they use rennet from either fungal or bacterial sources. And, advances in genetic engineering processes means the needed enzymes may be made using genetically altered micro-organisms (an improvement, but it doesn't sound much better to me).

Other substances may also be added during the cheese making process including calcium chloride, potassium nitrate, dyes, mold spores and bacteria. It's all a part of creating certain flavors like Roquefort (those blue veins are actually molds). Another issue is how the milk used is extracted from animals and whether it's been pasteurized...so there's a lot to consider.

I do have to say that cheese (and all dairy products including yogurt) is a source of protein, calcium, zinc, and vitamin B12. But remember that cheese is also a major source of saturated fat, which can lead to high cholesterol, increased risks of heart disease and strokes. Cheese like all animal derived proteins contains no carbohydrate or fiber, and is a very poor source of iron. So, take the information and make your own choice about cheese and dairy products.

HEAVY METALS

Heavy metal toxins have become known to cause health problems, especially since the industrial revolution. Heavy metals are everywhere...the water we drink, the foods we eat, the air we breathe, our daily household cleaners, our cookware and our other daily tools. Because it has a density at least five times that of water, heavy metal cannot be metabolized by the body. What that means is that it's not just any one source of metal, but the gradual and inevitable build up inside you that can lead to problems including impaired mental functions, decreased energy, nervous system, kidneys, lungs and other organ functions. So, it's important to be aware of the varied sources and look for ways to decrease your overall exposure in an effort to maintain your good health. Check out Fact File O for a list of metals, their typical sources and symptoms that could mean heavy metal poisoning.

MOLDS, MYCOTOXINS AND BACTERIA

Mold is one of those things we often have no idea is in our home and in the air we breathe until it's too late. Many molds cause allergic reactions and respiratory problems. And a few molds, in the right conditions, produce "mycotoxins," poisonous substances that can make people ill. Molds are found in virtually every environment and can be detected year round...indoors and outdoors. However, we're primarily going to be focusing on the molds that grow on your food items. Remember when you cleaned out your kitchen and got rid of things that could have mold...even if you didn't see it?

I know you tend to think of mold growing in the dark, moist, warm temperatures they prefer, but it can grow at refrigerator temperatures to. And, molds also tolerate salt and sugar better than most other food invaders. That's why you can get mold growing on your refrigerated jams and jelly and cured, salty meats - ham, bacon, salami and bologna.

Visually you only see part of the mold on the surface of food...grey fur on forgotten leftovers, fuzzy green dots on bread, white dust on Cheddar, coin-size velvety circles on fruits, and furry growth on the surface of jellies. By the time your food shows heavy mold growth the "root" threads it grows from have invaded your food deeply. In dangerous molds, poisonous substances are often contained in and around these threads. In some cases, toxins may have spread throughout the food. So, what does that mean? If you have moldy food – throw it out...don't just cut off the mold and eat what's left. You may still be ingesting mold.

So, how can you control mold growth on your food? Cleanliness is vital...mold spores from affected food can build up in your refrigerator, dishcloths, and other cleaning utensils. That's why I created a list of tips to keep you and your kitchen as mold-free as possible...you may want to print up Detail Divas Fact File P and stick it on your fridge for easy reference.

I hope I haven't alarmed you too much with some of the information in this chapter. My goal is not to frighten you, but to be sure you have all the information you need so you can go out and make Healthy Tart choices that fit with your lifestyle. If you'd like more information on any of these topics...visit the Detail Divas Appendices first, and then check out more in-depth information on my website – www.TrishaStewart.com.

Chapter 7

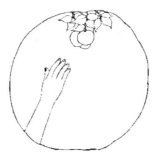

Claiming your Healthy Tartness

Whew! Well, you've made it this far...and that already shows your commitment to becoming the Healthy Tart you were meant to be. You've got all the tools and resources for your journey, now you just need to put it into a plan and put that plan into action. So, I'm going to be giving you a 30-day plan, some sample menus and a shopping list that will help get you started. Obviously you'll be customizing some things along the way to fit your tastes, budget and lifestyle...and that's great! Nothing is one size fits all...especially when you're looking at true lifestyle changes instead of some '30 days to thinner thighs' nonsense.

I know you're ready to get started, but before we get into the 30-day plan, I want to review some of the things you've learned along the way. That way, in case it's been a few days since you read chapter One...or even looked at the 10-steps...you'll get a quick refresher.

What have you learned??

What is a Healthy Tart? You in a few months...a woman who is ready for that long-term lifestyle change that means consistent nutritious foods and sensible exercise...as well as a bit of pampering to the outer body.

What and where is Eden? It's that idyllic place a Healthy Tart creates for herself that starts in the kitchen. It's a place where you've carved out a natural, non-polluted, energetic existence amidst the hectic (and sometimes toxic) work-a-day world around you.

How do you get to Eden? You take the 10-steps I've laid out for you...here's the list:

1. Clear the Decks – Getting rid of all the old, processed, unhealthy things
2. Equipment – Ensuring you have the right 'tools' for the job
3. Menu Planning – How to plan ahead to make life easy (and less tempting)
4. Shopping – What to buy, when to buy it and what to avoid
5. Time Management – How to fit Eden into your busy day
6. Goal Setting/Rewards – Setting yourself up for success

7. Exercise – Getting back on your feet, out the door and on the way

8. Detoxifying – Learning the benefits of detox and how to do it RIGHT

9. Body Treatments – Pampering your outside and staying natural

10. Putting it all together – How to juice and cook your way to health

What keeps you from Eden? It's all about facing the obstacles, recognizing the excuses and moving around them to keep on track.

What's good, what's bad and what's going on inside? You now have a better idea of all the things that go on inside you and why good food is so vital to your health. And, whether you wanted it or not...you've learned about what some of those bad foods (or the very ugly foods for that matter) are doing to your body. So, the choices are still up to you...but now you can make wise choices with the right information.

Lastly, and in many ways, most importantly...you've learned that change takes time. Forget about quick fixes, 10 minute exercises twice a week or the all or nothing approach. Unless you're battling a serious illness or disease, you're going to take this slowly...one step at a time. By the way...if you are battling a serious illness and you have NOT yet logged on to my website...please visit www.TrishaStewart.com so I can help you with a more personalized solution to your challenge. If that's not you...then remember we talked about 1% changes. Those little things you can do until they're habits, then you add the next one and then the next one. This is about setting yourself up for success instead of failure. I want your Healthy Tart lifestyle to become second nature to you. Forcing yourself to do a 180-degree turn around is NOT the way to make that happen. So as you review the steps and look over the 30-day plan, you can see your 'trouble spots'. That's where you can work on your first 1% changes.

Okay, now that you've got all of that refreshed in your mind, I know you're ready to take a look at this 30-day plan. I'm sure some of you have already done this...just couldn't wait to see what you had to do, could you? That's okay...I appreciate your enthusiasm. Remember that this 30-day plan includes a safe, gentle detoxification that you'll need to follow to get your system cleaned out and ready to run at optimum performance. Now if you have special needs or feel you cannot complete the 30-day plan, I urge you to log onto the website and connect with me and my team so we can create a personalized approach for you that addresses your specific situation. So, let's get started!!

The Healthy Tart's 30-Day Plan to Reach Eden

The 30-Day Plan is broken down into 5 sections. This plan is very doable...NO starvation...no constant hunger...no feeling faint. Each section carefully prepares you for the next phase and ultimately for getting your health and vitality back for keeps.

The 30-day Plan breaks down as follows:
- o   7 days – gentle detox
- o   5 days – light food
- o   2 days- juicing
- o   7 days – light food
- o   9 days – light food with introduction of certain other foods

A few notes to keep in mind during the next 30-days
- I have allowed light frying of foods, but remember to be careful how you fry or sauté. Use broths and other liquids or the smallest amounts of approved oils.
- Eat organic wherever possible
- The foods are vegetarian because they will be less taxing on the body systems and organs and will help to raise the Ph or alkalinity...thus flushing the body systems and organs.

- I have tried to create a program with a lot of variety and different foods for you to try, but don't feel you have to eat things you don't enjoy. You can focus on wholesome vegetable and bean soup, a juice, oats or muesli...but vary the ingredients and at least try a few new things.

- Try and be a bit more adventurous with the evening meal particularly at the weekend when you have time, experiment with different herbs, spices, vegetables etc and be creative. Feed more than your body...feed your soul.

- If you wish to swap your lunch for your evening meal this is okay and actually better for you.

- Check your bowels. They should be moving at least once a day...preferably more. If things are not 'moving', increase your fluids or visit my website (www.TrishaStewart.com).   And,   for   a   quick reference...revisit Chapter Three.

- Your urine will probably be quite colored and smelly for a day or so, but this will clear.

- You may go through what we term a "healing crisis" whereby you may get headaches, nausea and maybe a little feverish, and get facial or body spots. This will only last for a maximum of 48 hours. It's just your body adjusting to the changes and trying to eliminate toxins out of every orifice.   If this does happen increase your fluid intake and rest when possible. The best time to start your 30-day plan is over a weekend when you are not working, by Monday you will be raring to go.

- Remember, this is not like any of the quick fix detox plans. This is a way of eating that you can always come back to and should in the long term. I do not propose any quick fix...that is merely sticking a small band aid over a major wound. I am talking lifelong health, so these changes to your eating can be implemented every day or your life. This is a healthy way to eat long term. But I do know the other foods will creep in so you can always come back to Step 8 or sooner if you begin to lose the vitality that you will gain over the next 30 days and beyond.

- At this stage we will use products that will enhance the cleansing and healing process rather than add vitamins and minerals. The main reason is that your gut will probably be compromised at this stage and not absorbing as well as it should and will be in a short time. And, as long as you're eating a good, balanced organic diet...I don't believe in long term use of supplements anyway. However, you may find benefits with these supplements:

    1. Acidophilus culture. Lactobacillus acidophilus in capsule or powdered form will add good

bacteria to the intestines and bowel and help in controlling the bad bacteria.

2. Milk Thistle, great for supporting the liver
3. Omega 3,6,9 from seed oil for helping to reduce inflammation and calm the nervous system
4. MSM (methylsulfonymethane) a great sulphur rich cleanser for the whole system

- Cut out the following products from your diet:
    1. Yeast in bread, rolls, pizza, gravy powders, marmite, etc.
    2. Wheat in flour (unless unrefined), cereals, readymade products
    3. Cut out all sugar, that which you add and that which is already added. Including biscuits, cakes, chocolate, sweets, ice creams, puddings, chewing gum, sweeteners and anything that says it is sugar free but has a sweetener in it.
    4. Fruit consumption is to be pears and apples(for first seven days) only (no dried fruits in muesli or eaten on their own)
    5. No added salt or very minimal rock salt only
    6. No takeaways, ready meals, fast foods, etc.
    7. All meat, game and poultry, fish, eggs
    8. Coffee, tea, hot chocolate, etc.

9. All dairy foods
10. Refined grains i.e. those not with the hull intact
11. All alcohol
12. Smoking (if possible PLEASE!)
13. Over the counter medicines
14. And, finally check with your doctor to make sure you are not being over-prescribed medication.

- Eat plenty of the following foods freely
  1. All vegetables/salads/herbs raw or cooked
     - Fresh vegetable juices anytime
     - Keep a pan of soup on the go for anytime
     - Have some crudités ready for nibbling or dipping into hummus, guacamole and other dips (I've included a few dip recipes)
  2. Nuts and seeds
  3. Pears, avocado, apples. Other fruits in season but limited for the first seven days
  4. Whole grains such as wholegrain rice, quinoa etc
  5. Sprouted beans, seeds etc.
  6. Breakfast oats, millet or quinoa

7. Tofu or other soya bean products (not ready made sausages/burgers etc as they will contain salt or other flavorings

8. Soya Yogurts. Milk

9. Nut milks or rice milk

10. Nut and seed butters

- Fluids to include

    1. Filtered spring or distilled water hot or cold

    2. Fruit or herbal teas

    3. Chinese Green teas

NOTE: Any of the menu items below that have an asterisk (*) means I have included the recipe in the following section.

Seven days - Gentle Detox

- Start each day with a pint of hot water with lemons and limes infused
- Mid-morning and mid-afternoon have crudités with a dip (mid-morning) and a handful of nuts and seeds (mid-afternoon) or in reverse according to what you fancy. Or, have a bowl of light vegetable soup.

Monday

Breakfast: *Healthy Tart porridge or *Healthy Tart muesli topped with apples and pears, stewed or raw

Lunch: Healthy Tart Veggie Salad: Mixed leaf salad with sprouts, nuts and seeds, avocado, grated beetroot, celery, courgette, grated carrot and cherry tomatoes. Make a dressing from olive oil, lemon/lime juice, crushed garlic plus any herbs you may favor, shake it all up in a jar.

Dinner: Enjoy lots of different vegetables and beans to serve with whole grain rice or quinoa, may be made into a curry, chili (use fresh chili if possible far nicer flavor than powder) or a casserole

Tuesday

Breakfast: Stewed pears/apples and natural soya yoghurt flavored with nutmeg, vanilla, topped with nuts and seeds or homemade muesli

Lunch: *Simple homemade carrot and coriander soup with a mixed leaf salad & sprouts

Dinner: *Tofu and bean burgers with mixed vegetables selection and homemade sweet potato wedges and a dip of your choice from the recipe section.

Wednesday

Breakfast: Breakfast as usual or *buckwheat pancakes with stewed fruit folded inside plus a juice from the recipes

Lunch: Quinoa and veggie salad with a *spicy dressing

Dinner: *Provencal stew, rice pasta or polenta with a green salad to include baby leaf spinach, parsley, lambs lettuce, beet greens or whatever you fancy

Thursday

Breakfast: *Lentil patties with lightly sautéed tomatoes plus a juice from any of the recipes

Lunch: Homemade soup with a mixed salad of sprouts and leaves

Dinner: *Poached Tofu in a Thai sauce, garlic potatoes, steamed spinach or kale, carrots and fresh peas

Friday

Breakfast: Healthy Tart porridge Healthy Tart muesli with apples and pears

Lunch: Wholegrain rice and root vegetable with a dressing (cold or hot)

Dinner: *Bean casserole topped with potatoes; serve with green vegetables in season

Saturday

Breakfast: Apples and pears with natural soya yoghurt and nutmeg

Lunch: Baked sweet potato with ratatouille

Dinner: *Vegetable paella (can be used as it is or to stuff peppers, aubergines or any other vegetable you can stuff)

Sunday

Breakfast: Sauté potatoes, mushrooms, tomatoes and onions

Lunch: Large green salad with a selection of other vegetables homemade coleslaw

Dinner: *Nut roast with red onion gravy, green vegetables, roasted roots

I realize this may not sound like much of a detox, but believe me you will have missed your bread, sugar and...for meat eaters...your flesh foods. But, you will feel a whole lot

better, probably lost a few pounds and will have renewed energy. Keep going. Did I hear anyone say they had not had indigestion this week and bowel movements were good? Check these daily!

Five Days - Light Food

Ok so you have now completed seven really important days, seven days that will enhance the rest of your life. The next five days will remain very similar but with the inclusion of other fruits which will be juiced or eaten whole plus a two day only weekend of juicing. Try to eat with the seasons so whatever fruit is available but avoid grapes and banana and if using melon do not have it with other fruits, eat it alone. Keep these pointers in mind:

- Keep up with the fluids and snacks as before.
- If you can grow some sprouts this week, even if it is only alfalfa that would be great for your juices and of course added to any other foods.
- Don't forget to drink a pint of hot water with lemon and limes as soon as you rise from your bed and to drink at least two liters more during the day.

Monday

Breakfast: Make a breakfast juice of apples, carrot, celery, parsley, spinach, pineapple and a little natural soya yoghurt if you like the texture smooth.

Lunch: Homemade vegetable soup with beans and a leafy salad

Dinner: *Red peppers stuffed with spicy vegetables served with green vegetables or salad

Tuesday

Breakfast: Juice as before with maybe some variation according to what you enjoy and what is in season

Lunch: Homemade vegetable soup with beans and a green salad

Dinner: Tofu and vegetable Thai curry with wholegrain rice and raita

Wednesday

Breakfast: Oats with apples and pears or a juice or both if you feel hungry

Lunch: *Tabouleh with a green salad

Dinner: *Parsnip and carrot risotto with steamed spinach or other green vegetable or salad

Thursday

Breakfast: Juice and Healthy Tart porridge or Healthy Tart
            muesli
Lunch: Beetroot cooked and sliced, red onion sliced
            thinly, crumbled walnut sat on top of a large leafy
            salad, all the herb leaves as well as usual lettuce
            leaves and herbs
Dinner: * Lentil dhal and roasted garlic with steamed
            green vegetables and wild rice

Friday
Breakfast: Juice as before

Lunch: Large bowl of homemade soup with a salad
Dinner: Parsnip, chickpeas with onions, *chili and ginger
            sauce, quinoa, and raita

Two Days - Juicing

Because by now your body should be working a lot more
efficiently, your kidneys, bladder, bowels and liver should be
much more active, what a great job you have done! But now
brace yourselves for juicing. If you can't manage to just juice
please add in some soups instead of or as well as. I am not
letting you off the hook here, but if you REALLY cannot face it
please go to two of the days the previous week and repeat
the menu but I have to tell you if you are on a weight loss
track this will certainly help to drop a few more pounds.

You will need to relax and have a chill out weekend. Ensure you have scheduled this in, you have had plenty of time to do so, no excuses, and this is your life! It's a great time to do a salt scrub and an Epsom salt bath (not if you have high blood pressure though please), or a gentle bath in some essential oils. Revisit Step Ten on skin brushing...have you tried this yet?

Okay, here's the basic juice program. You will have five juices daily, plus masses of filtered water and soups...but only vegetable soups. No grains or beans to be added to the soup. Note that some of the juice recipes are for one person, please increase accordingly for more people.

Day One:
On rising have a pint of hot water with lemon/lime slices. Then make the following juices (with your juicer...remember not a blender or smoothie maker).

8am juice	Two apples, stick of celery, handful of spinach or kale, ¼ pineapple, ½ ripe avocado
11am juice	Two apples, Medium carrot, handful mixed leaves (kale, spinach, parsley) ½ medium sized beetroot, ¼ lemon, ginger to taste, alfalfa sprouts

2pm juice	Similar to the 11am juice but add in anything that you feel like to go with it, maybe avocado or cucumber or broccoli or some other herbs
5pm juice	Two apples, one pear, ½ pineapple, handful of greens, stick of celery, ¼ avocado, chunk courgette
8pm	Make this a smoothie using soya natural yoghurt, nice and relaxing for the end of the day. Some fruits of your choice including half of a banana, half avocado.
	Before bed if you feel like it stew some apples and add cinnamon.

Day Two:
Repeat the same idea on Sunday but have a supper of chunky vegetable soup with beans. You should be raring to go on Monday so up you get, pint of hot water with lemons/limes, have your mid morning and mid afternoon snacks as usual.

7 Days - Light Food
For the next week, you will have a mixture of the previous two weeks. Keep in mind all of the previous notes about water intake and starting each day with a pint of hot water

with the lemons/limes infusion. You can change up the menu a bit to suit your tastes.

Monday

Breakfast: Fruit and natural soya yoghurt with nuts and seeds or a juice of your choice or both

Lunch: Big chunky soup with side salad

Dinner: *Simple root veggie hotpot with green vegetables and homemade potato wedges and a dip of your choice from the recipe section

Tuesday

Breakfast: Juice

Lunch: Spicy lentil and bean with a leafy salad

Dinner: Tofu, vegetable and cashew nut sir fry with a *ginger and chili sauce, serve with wholegrain rice or quinoa

Wednesday

Breakfast: Healthy Tart porridge or muesli with fresh fruit and/or a juice

Lunch: Large salad with lots of different vegetables/leaves, tomatoes, basil or other herb dressing, avocado, nuts and seeds and sprouts and olives

Dinner: *No meat shepherd's pie with carrots and green vegetables

Thursday

Breakfast: Juice and *Tofu scramble

Lunch: Chunky soup and salad

Dinner: Vegetable and chickpea curry with wholegrain rice or quinoa and raita

Friday

Breakfast: Healthy Tart porridge or muesli with fruit and/or juice

Lunch: Sliced avocado, thinly sliced onions, sliced tomatoes, sliced cucumber, topped with hummus and olives

Dinner: Roasted root salad with whole garlic, marinated tofu and homemade coleslaw

Saturday

Breakfast: Potato cakes, mushrooms, tomatoes, onions

Lunch: Jacket potato with a spice bean filling or ratatouille

Dinner: *Pasta with a red pepper sauce and a huge salad

Sunday

Breakfast: Juice, Healthy Tart porridge or muesli

Lunch: *Stuffed peppers

Dinner: Lentil Dhal with fried vegetable rice and steamed
            spinach or other green vegetable

Hopefully this week has worked wonders for your digestive system and your energy will have increased.

9 Days - Light food & Extras

The following and last seven days of your 30-day plan will include a couple of little extras... not much though, so don't get too excited. Instead, be excited about how you are feeling...your renewed energy, clear skin and eyes. I bet your nails have grown also. Check in with yourself to see how you really feel and what has changed and give yourself a pat on the back for doing so well.

The following seven days will include all of the foods you have eaten before but you may have some oat cakes, rice cakes, corn crackers. I will do a "pick and mix" of the recipes so that you eat a variety of beans, grains, legumes, tofu, etc. Saturday and Sunday will include foods that you may have periodically during the weeks ahead such a tortilla wraps or soda bread, sourdough, flatbreads etc. But please be aware they may upset your tummy so don't not eat too much.

Breakfast each day
Healthy Tart Porridge or muesli with fruit/or homemade juice.

Snacks each day

You can now include a couple of oat cakes with some hummus or guacamole or nuts/seeds or a bowl of light vegetable soup.

Monday

Lunch: Large salad with grated root vegetables, avocado, walnuts, cherry tomatoes and a dressing

Dinner: *Teriyaki style tofu with Asian noodles

Tuesday

Lunch: Homemade soup with salad and corn crackers

Dinner: Chickpea curry served with wholegrain rice

Wednesday

Lunch: Tabouleh served on a bed or leaves

Dinner: Tofu Thai style with wild rice and steamed greens

Thursday

Lunch: Jacket Potato stuffed with chili, ratatouille or other favorite

Dinner: Provencal stew with rice pasta or polenta and green vegetables or salad

Friday

Lunch: Homemade soup, salad and oatcakes

Dinner: Tofu Burgers, potato wedges, salad and a dip of
             your choice from the recipe section

Saturday
Lunch: Avocado salad
Dinner: Carrot and parsnip risotto with green beans

Sunday
Lunch: Potato rostis with dips and a salad
Dinner: Nut roast with a red onion sauce, green vegetables
             and roast potatoes

From here on:

- Once every other day you can include any yeast free
  bread, preferably rye flour or sourdough, tortilla
  wraps, oat cakes, rice cakes (all sugar, yeast and
  preservative free so probably best to make them or
  purchase them from a very good supplier)
- Vary the vegetables raw and cooked, the grains and
  pulses see shopping list or the good bad and ugly
- Carnivores please try to keep to a minimum of meat,
  poultry, game and fish, after the next seven days you
  may include a little more but hopefully you will have
  enjoyed the vegetarian foods so much your tastes will
  have changed forever.

At the end of these 30 days you're going to feel amazing...more energy, more vibrant, you'll have likely lost some weight and you'll have a real working idea of how and what you should be eating every day. Following are a few tools to make your journey to Eden a little easier.

First, I've included a 7-day journal you can use to track your eating and exercise and especially, how you're feeling as you work through the 30-day plan. You can also access our online journal if you prefer the electronic approach to journaling. Second, I've included some recipes for many of the new dishes I'd like you to try and to help you learn how to cook in a healthier way. And, to be sure you don't get stranded in your kitchen without the right foods; I've provided you an easy access shopping list. Remember, you don't have to make yourself eat foods you dislike...but this is a great opportunity to introduce your pallet to some wonderful, new tastes. And, just like our journal, you can access the shopping list online...which makes it easy for you to customize it for your tastes.

Recipes for the 30-day Plan

Healthy Tart Porridge

This can be a simple cupful of oats to 3 or 4 cups of water or a mix of water and some kind of milk. Put in a small pan, just bring to simmer for a few minutes, add more fluid if necessary. It will depend on the oats as to how much fluid. You can make millet or quinoa porridge in exactly the same way but may need to vary the fluid

Or make a mix of oats, millet and quinoa.

You can add to this the following:

1. Pure vanilla essence or a vanilla pod
2. Nutmeg
3. Cinnamon
4. Nuts and Seeds, ground or whole
5. Fresh stewed fruit
6. A little soya yoghurt

Oatcakes

350gm of fine oatmeal or coarse if you like a rustic oatcake

1 tsp. of good quality rock salt

150ml pint boiling water

50 ml of olive oil, walnut or other oil (may need to check consistency and add more) you can also use Tahini, Nut butter or any Vegan Butter that will melt.

Pinch of bicarbonate of soda

Mix everything together and turn out onto a board, knead and roll out into two big rounds. Make some cuts across to form triangles and bake on a tray which has been oiled. Bake in a cool oven of around 150C/300F or gas mark 2 for about one hour, do not overcook or they will be too hard.

Healthy Tart Muesli

1 cup of each of rice flakes and millet. Add chopped nuts, sunflower seeds, sesame seeds, pumpkin seeds and flax seeds. Soak in soya or rice milk for half an hour or less -if you like the mixture a little dry then top with soya (natural) yoghurt.

Rice bread

125 grams (4oz) rice flakes, 1 cup mineral water, 125gms pea or lentil flour, 125gms ground almonds or brazil nuts, 125gsm kholrabi, grated, 2 tablespoon sesame seed oil or olive oil, 1 tablespoon tapioca flour or arrowroot, 1 teaspoon cream of tartar, 1/2 teaspoon bicarbonate of soda. Preheat oven to 150 (300) or gas 2, pour water onto rice flakes, leave to soak for 5 minutes, mix all ingredients and bake in a lined 2lb loaf tin.

Savory millet, lentil and brazil nut loaf

125gms millet, 125gsm green lentils, sprouted, 1 cup vegetable stock or mineral water, 1 tablespoon tapioca flour, 125gsm roughly chopped brazil nuts, 2 sticks celery, 1 tablespoon fresh sage.

Preheat oven to 150 (310) or gas 3, cook millet and lentils in the stock or mineral water and mix with rest of ingredients, oil loaf tin or deep pie dish and press mixture well in, bake for 45 minutes or until top of loaf is brown and firm to touch.

Simple carrot and coriander soup (use other vegetables and herbs in to create your own Homemade Soup)

Use 1lb of carrots to 1½ pints of yeast free vegetable stock (cube will do but use low salt one).

Put a small amount of olive oil into base of large pan, put in one chopped onion, clove of garlic and sweat (on low with lid on) for a few minutes. Add chopped carrots plus a large chopped potato plus one leek (optional). Pour on stock, bring to boil then turn down and simmer until cooked. Add fresh bunch of coriander

When cooled I like to blend three parts and leave some chunky bits in, but this is your choice, blend all or none if preferred.

Tofu and Bean Burgers

Makes 6-8

1 medium onion, peeled and chopped

1 large peeled garlic clove or to taste

1 medium carrot, peeled and coarsely grated (about 60g

prepared weight)

420g can 'no-salt no-sugar' red kidney beans, drained and rinsed in a colander under cold running water or a mix of other beans

220g pack smoked or natural tofu, drained

75g/ cup sunflower seeds

1 small bunch parsley (about 20g)

2 tsp organic wheat and yeast free vegetable bouillon powder

Preheat the oven to 220C/430F Gas Mark 7. Line a large baking tray with baking parchment Place all the ingredients in a food processor and blend for roughly do not puree.   If you don't have a food processor, crumble or mash the tofu and beans and add to the other ingredients.

 Grab a handful of mixture and form into a ball and place on the baking tray. Press with fingertips to make a burger shape, how many you will get depends on the size burger you would like.

Bake for 25 minutes, do not overcook, these are great hot or cold or served with a creamy sauce.

Buckwheat Pancakes

This is a basic recipe; you may like to play around with different ingredients to make this work for you. They will not be as light as the usual pancakes as you are using different flours and egg replacer

1 heaped cup buckwheat flour

2 + teaspoons baking powder

Pinch of rock salt

1 cup soy milk, rice milk or almond milk

1 teaspoon pure vanilla essence

2 Tablespoons ground almonds or finely chopped walnuts

For variety you can add nut butters such as almond or seeds

butter such as Tahini (sesame) when blending the wet

ingredients

Beat it all together and ladle into a frying pan which has hot

olive or sunflower oil in it.

Provencal Stew

1 large onion, chopped

Garlic and olive oil, to taste

1 large aubergine/eggplant, cut into cubes (salted, drained,

and blotted dry if desired)

2 red peppers, sliced

3 large tomatoes, seeded and chopped

2 courgette/zucchini, chopped

Salt and pepper to taste

Herbes de Provence Dried which should be a mix of

Rosemary, Basil, Marjoram, Savory, and Thyme. I also like

to put in fresh Basil it has such a wonderful smell and taste,

add towards the end.

- Sauté onion and garlic in olive oil
- Add the aubergine/eggplant and fry a few minutes.

- Add the peppers, tomatoes and zucchini.
- Add herbs to taste.
- Let cook over medium-low heat for 30 minutes, stirring occasionally.

Serve hot as a main dish, or cold as a side dish.

This is a very handy recipe as you can stuff it into jacket (sweet or white) potato, or stuff any vegetable that is "stuffable."

Lentil Rissoles

Cup dry lentils, (red/green/brown) cooked in 2 cups water
1 cup carrots, shredded or finely diced
1 medium onion, finely chopped
1 cup red or green pepper finely diced
1 courgette/zucchini finely diced
2 cups medium/fine oats
1/4 cup extra virgin olive oil
3/4 cup tomato paste
1 tablespoon Italian seasoning

- Bring water to boil and put lentils in, bring back to simmer for about 15 minutes or until just soft.
- Sauté the onions in a frying/sauté pan until they look translucent, do not brown
- Add peppers and courgette/zucchini cook until just softening

- Put the ingredients in a bowl and add the lentils and bind together
- Shape them into rolls, rounds, squares or whatever suits you.

You can add spices to these for a change and try different vegetables such as celery or spinach, sweet potato mashed with the lentil mixture, they are great hot or cold.

Poached Tofu and Thai Sauce

2 Sweet red chilies seeded and chopped

1 lemon grass stalk chopped

1inch piece of ginger root, peeled and chopped finely

2 Kaffir Lime Leaves

1 bunch fresh coriander (cilantro)

1 tsp ground coriander

(if the above ingredients are not available use dried, it will not be as nice and you will have to blend to taste)

1 pack of Tofu, (plain, smoked or herb) cubed or sliced

- Put all the above ingredients (except the Tofu) into a food processor or use a pestle and mortar and blend
- Add 400ml of coconut milk to the above and mix together

- Place in a frying or sauté pan and add the Tofu and simmer so that the ingredients can come together in flavor, about 20 minutes or more if preferred.

Bean Casserole

2 large onions sliced

Little olive oil

2 cloves garlic diced (or to taste)

1" piece of ginger sliced or diced

4 Tomatoes sliced

½ Courgette/zucchini sliced

4 Tbl Tahini

500ml vegetable stock from yeast free boullion or homemade stock

Mixed beans such as Haricot, Kidney, Flageolet, Butter (cooked) if using tinned ensure sugar and salt free and rinse thoroughly

2 tsp mixed dried herbs such as Italian or Provence

1 Large Sweet Potato sliced

Fresh herbs to dress

- In a large sauté pan, put a little olive oil and sauté the sliced onions till translucent
- Add the garlic and ginger, sauté for a minute or two
- Add the tomatoes and courgettes
- Add the beans

- Mix the tahini, herbs and vegetable stock and add to the mixture, do not make it too wet at this stage
- Put into a casserole dish
- Place the sweet potato on top
- Bake in the oven on 170c/325f gas 3 for about an hour

You can leave it all in the sauté pan, put the potato on top and simmer with a lid on, baked in the oven is nicer though

You may need to add a little stock if the casserole gets to look dry

Vegetable paella (fast version)

Portion of cooked wholegrain rice

1 large sliced onion

1 clove garlic sliced or diced

1 stick celery sliced

1 carrot cut into sticks

1 red or green pepper cut into slices

1 courgette/zucchini cut into sticks

Mange tout left whole or sliced

Yeast free vegetable stock

- In a large flat frying pan sauté some garlic, onions and celery in olive oil for 5 minutes
- Add sticks of carrot, peppers, courgettes, mange tout or any vegetables you like.
- Add the rice

- Add the stock to taste, not too wet
- Add pine nuts, broken cashew nuts, olives and serve with green salad.

The above paella ingredients are ideal to stuff peppers, aubergines and any other 'stuffable' vegetables.

If you want to make the longer version, add uncooked risotto rice, about 1 cup to the onions, garlic and celery mix, then add the vegetables and ladle in the stock so that the rice can cook, this is a little time consuming but very nice although I do find risotto rice very starchy compared to wholegrain, so not ideal.

Nut Roast

1tbs extra-virgin olive oil

3 cups of mixed nuts, ground or finely chopped

12 oz tomatoes, blanched, peeled & chopped or tinned

1 large onion

1 clove garlic diced

1/4lb fresh mushrooms, chopped

1/2 tsp dried basil and dried oregano or other mixed herbs to taste

1 - 1/2 cups of cooked millet or quinoa

Directions

- Preheat oven to 425F (220C) gas 7
- Lightly oil a loaf tin

- Sauté the onion and garlic in a little olive oil until the onion is translucent
- Place these in a mixing bowl and add the rest of the ingredients
- Turn the mixture into the prepared loaf tin, smoothing the surface with the back of a spoon. Place the tin in oven and bake for 30-40 minutes

Serve with an onion gravy made from sliced onions sautéed in olive oil, 1 1/2 cups of vegetable stock, 1 tbsp tomato paste, 1 tsp mustard, bring to a simmer until cooked.

Tabouleh

1 cup of bulgur wheat

1 ½ cups of boiling water

3 tbsp lemon juice

1 clove garlic grated or crushed in a pestle and mortar

Bunch of fresh mint chopped or ½ tsp dried

¾ tbsp olive oil

4/6 spring onions chopped (use the green if nice)

3 tomatoes diced

1 small cucumber diced

½ cup of olives if liked

Bunch parsley some chopped some left for garnish

- Combine the bulgar wheat and water, stir and let sit for 30 minutes to re-hydrate
- Stir after the 30 minutes to check there is no moisture, if there is drain off
- Add lemon juice, garlic and oil
- Add the remaining ingredients and stir

This is nice if left to sit for a while so that the flavors can combine.

Parsnip and Carrot Risotto

1 ½ cups of dry rice (check with the paella recipe for the fast or slow version)

1 large sliced onion

1 clove garlic diced

2/3 carrots cut into sticks

1/2 parsnips cut into sticks

1 liter or more of yeast free vegetable stock

Bunch Fresh coriander chopped (or other fresh herbs)

Olive oil

- Sauté the onion in a little olive oil with the garlic
- Add the uncooked rice (if doing the slow version)
- Add the parsnip and carrots

- Ladle in the stock to allow the rice and vegetables to cook in a little of the liquid, adding more as ingredients begin to dry
- Just towards the end add the fresh coriander or other herbs

If doing the fast version and using cooked rice, add this just before the vegetables are cooked and then add the stock to taste do not make too wet. This does not hurt to simmer slowly until you are ready to eat.

Red Lentil Dhal

Olive oil

1 tsp garlic, crushed

1 tsp each fresh chili and ginger, finely chopped and mixed

2 tsp powdered turmeric

1 tsp garam masala

1 tsp ground coriander

2 tbsp fresh coriander, finely chopped

1 cinnamon stick

1 tsp mustard

1 large whole tomato, diced finely

1 medium onion, diced finely

2 sticks celery, diced finely

800ml water

225gms red lentils, washed well

- Heat the oil in a saucepan with a thick base

- Add garlic, chili, ginger and spices (except fresh coriander) and herbs, mustard, tomato, onion and celery.
- Fry for about 10 minutes until well blended.
- Add the water and bring to the boil
- Stir the lentils in and cook on a low heat for about half an hour, until the lentils are soft, stirring occasionally.

You may need to add a little stock or water if the dhal becomes dry. If you have time place a couple of bulbs of garlic in the oven and roast for half an hour, take out and press the juicy roasted garlic and add to the dhal, some chopped almonds on top are nice and also the fresh coriander.

This is a good side dish for a vegetable curry, good on its own with some homemade spicy onion koftas

Stir Fried Greens, Ginger and Oyster Sauce

  1lb Chinese greens, Pak Choy and Baby Spinach.

  1 tablespoons walnut oil

  1 tablespoon sesame oil

  1" sliced fresh ginger

  1 fresh red chili sliced

  4 spring onions

  2 tablespoons oyster sauce (no added sugar)

  ¼ yeast free stock cube make up a with a little water

Juice of ½ lemon, black pepper

- Blanche Pak Choy for 1 minute in boiling water and drain.
- In large wok fry ginger and onions in oils, add rest of ingredients, add oyster sauce and stock cube and lemon juice.
- If you want more sauce add water and thicken with potato starch.
- Serve with rice noodles or rice or quinoa.

Raita relish, dip or condiment

200 ml soya yoghurt

1/8 tsp cumin powder

Pinch paprika

½ cup cucumber finely diced

1 tsp. finely crushed coriander leaves

- Whisk the yoghurt
- Add the other ingredients
- Garnish with fresh coriander

To ring the changes try using finely diced tomato, onion, cooked potato, blanched shredded spinach or other vegetable you like.

Simple Root Vegetable Hotpot

- Sauté/sweat a chopped onion and garlic in a pan

- add a variety of chopped vegetables (about 1 1/2 lb), tin tomatoes, herbs and a half pint of water with some yeast free stock with a little tomato puree, simmer gently or put in the oven.

Make sure that the hot pot does not dry; you may need a little more water depending on vegetables used. Add some cooked lentils or other pulses/beans to make a more substantial meal

Tofu, vegetable and cashew nut stir fry (serve with rice or other grain)

1 pack Tofu, cubed

1 large onion sliced

1 garlic clove diced

1 inch piece of ginger root diced or grated

2 fresh sweet chillis, de-seeded and chopped finely

A mix of thinly sliced vegetables such as carrot, green or red peppers, celery, zucchini/courgette, mange tout or fresh peas (any you fancy)

Cashew Nuts

- Heat a small amount of olive oil in a wok or large frying pan
- Add tofu and lightly fry till golden brown, then remove.
- Add the onion and garlic, chili and ginger, sauté for a few minutes

- Put in a mixture of thinly sliced carrots, green pepper, ginger, celery etc and sauté for 1 min to mix flavors
- Add some cashews
- Add a little yeast free stock; put in the tofu and sauté all vegetables until they are as soft as you would like them.

No meat Shepherd's Pie

110g (4oz) brown lentils

900g (2lbs) potatoes, roughly chopped

3 tbsp olive oil

3-5 tbsp soya milk

8oz onions or leeks sliced

4oz carrots, small slices

4oz parsnips, small slices

8oz mushrooms, roughly chopped

3-4 sticks celery, sliced

2 tbsp tomato puree

225g (8oz) chopped tomatoes fresh or tinned

1tbsp soy sauce

1/8tsp rosemary

1tsp dried oregano

- Cook the lentils in stock or water until they are tender (about 1 hour).

- Cook the potatoes in boiling salted water. When tender, drain and mash with the milk to obtain creamy (not sloppy) mashed potatoes. Season to taste.
- Meanwhile sauté the onions, celery, carrots and parsnips with a small amount of olive oil, until almost tender. If they are slow in cooking, add a bit of water, cover and cook until the carrots are tender.
- Add the mushrooms and continue to cook until they are softening, then add the lentils, tomatoes, tomato puree, oregano and rosemary and cook for a few more minutes. Season to taste with soy sauce and salt and pepper.
  Spread out in an ovenproof dish. Cover with mashed potatoes about 2cm thick. Bake at 200C (375F, gas 5) for 30-40 minutes

Tofu Scramble

This is one of those simple recipes to make with a variation to suit so try your own.

The basis is 1 pack Tofu

1 small onion finely diced

A little diced garlic

Red pepper, courgette, zucchini, whatever you have diced

A little turmeric or cumin or other spices or herbs that you like

A little olive oil to fry in

- Drain, cube and crumble the Tofu
- Sauté off the onion, garlic, spices or herbs (if fresh leave till last)
- Add your choice of vegetables cook till you like the consistency

Quick Bean Salad - add some mixed salad leaves and rice or other grain

Mix a variety of dried, cooked beans such as kidney, borlotti, black eye, flageolet with some lightly steamed French, broad or runner beans and mixed fresh herbs, olive oil and lemon/lime juice. You can buy tinned for emergencies but ensure sugar and salt free.

Adding curry spices to this makes a change

Quick Rice and lentil salad - add some mixed salad leaves

Cook rice and lentils according to type, cool and add a
variety of chopped vegetables such as pepper, cucumber,
spring onions, celery, sweet corn, carrots, fennel, *anything
you like* and stir in some olive oil, lemon/lime juice with a
few nuts and seeds and selected fresh herbs (plenty of
them) Or you could use spices mixed in a little olive oil (a
curry paste)

Simple stir fry

One dessert teaspoon olive oil
Variety of vegetables i.e. broccoli, courgettes, peppers,
mange tout (or sugar snap) bean sprouts, carrots - anything
you fancy or have in. Chopped or sliced.
Sauté/sweat a chopped onion and clove of garlic. Add
Grated ginger.
Add vegetables and cook to your liking, add a little water
and some Tamari/soya sauce if liked.

Vary all the ingredients to create other tastes e.g. instead of
ginger add mixed herbs, black olives.

Roasted Root Salad
Delicious hot but also good when cold and eaten with rice, quinoa, millet or other grain

2lb parsnips, peeled and trimmed, cut into thick chips.
1lb carrots, peeled and trimmed, cut into thick chips.
4 tablespoon olive oil.

14oz cooked beetroot peeled and chopped.

One half onion finely diced.

2 teaspoon chopped fresh herbs.

Gas 6 / 200c/390f electric.

Place parsnips and carrots in a lightly oiled pan (using olive oil), then lightly brush them over with more olive oil plus a few tablespoons of water to prevent the vegetables drying out. Cook for about 45 minutes turning halfway so that they get all crispy.

When cooked remove to a bowl and add the beetroot, onion and herbs, mix and serve.

Quick Mixed Bean Chili - can be served with rice or other grain and a green salad

You can use tinned beans but ensure they are sugar free, drained and washed.

Please use carrots and carrot juice if tomatoes are not allowed and omit tomato puree

Sweat off 1 large onion and 2/3 cloves of garlic in a little olive oil add a pinch or more of chili powder, 1 tablespoon of tomato puree and paprika and cook for 1-2 minutes. Add tinned tomatoes, beans and mixed vegetables (courgette, carrots, peppers etc.) and cook until tender

Quick Cashew Nut and Vegetable Pilaf - good hot or cold

Sauté 1 large onion and 2/3 cloves of garlic for about 5 minutes, add celery and peppers, brown rice 300gms uncooked weight, stir, add 1.5 pints of vegetable stock and bring to boil, turn down and simmer for about 20/25minutes until rice is cooked and liquid is absorbed. Stir in 4oz of chopped cashew nuts and some fresh parsley.

Vegetable Tikka

Choose vegetables to suit, ones that will cook easily or part cook before marinating. chop, slice or cube i.e. courgette/zucchini, aubergine, sweet potato, peppers, tomatoes, fennel, mushrooms etc.

1 medium onion, 2 cloves, small piece ginger, 4 tablespoons soya yoghurt or vegetable oil, juice of ½ lemon, 2 fresh chilies, 2 teaspoons coriander seeds, 1 teaspoon cumin, ½ teaspoon turmeric powder, fresh 10 mint leaves, ¼ teaspoon garam massala.

Dry roast seeds and grind, grind spices and add to rest of ingredients leave overnight or for several hours to marinate and then fast cook under grill or griddle until crispy
Serve with lemon and salad leaves and rice.

Penne Pasta & Red Pepper Sauce

1 large red pepper and 1 onion for the sauce.

1lb pasta, 2 medium courgettes, 12 olives, 1 large onion, 2 cloves garlic, mixed fresh herbs (basil, marjoram, oregano,) 6 tablespoons olive oil, ½ grated bread roll (yeast free), soft green peppercorns and squeeze of lemon juice.

Cook pasta in boiling water. In a separate pan sauté large onion (chopped, diced medium), courgettes, chopped garlic. Add all the ingredients to the cooked pasta, add grated breadcrumbs and put into serving bowl.

For the sauce, sauté onions, add chopped peppers and ½ stock cube (yeast free), cover with water, bring to boil and simmer for 30 minutes, either mix in with or pour over pasta dish.

Serve with large mixed salad.

Hummus

12os chickpeas (soaked overnight), ¼ teaspoon ground cumin, 1 fresh chili, 1 clove garlic, 1 ½ tablespoons tahini, 4 tablespoon olive oil, 2 tablespoon lemon juice, pepper.

Boil chickpeas approx 1-1.5 hours till tender, drain saving a little of the water, blend with other ingredients in machine till smooth add water if you want a thinner mix.

Salad Dressings

Oriental

6 tablespoons olive oil, 2 teaspoons of lemon juice, 4
teaspoons soy sauce, ½ teaspoon grated root ginger put into
a jar and shake.

French

6 tablespoons olive oil, 2 tablespoons lemon juice, 2
tablespoons cider vinegar. Variations on the above could
include crushed garlic, balsamic vinegar, mustard and any
fresh herbs you may like. Shake it all in a jar or put into a
blender.

Soy Yoghurt

Take a tub of natural soya yoghurt and put in a blender with
a choice of any herbs or spices, this will make a dressing or
a dip for crudités. Whip in a blender

Sundried Tomato Dressing

100ml olive oil, 2tablespoons tomato puree or sun dried
tomatoes,
1 teaspoon cumin, allspice, oregano, marjoram and a little
cayenne pepper (vary any). Whizz in a blender

Stuffed Peppers

4 peppers (1 for each person, reduce the whole recipe if just catering for one)

1 tbsp. olive oil

1 small onion finely chopped

1 clove garlic, minced

1 tsp. oregano

1 tsp. basil

2 carrots cut into fine sticks

1 Zucchini/courgette cut into fine sticks

1 tomato, diced

½ cup pine nuts or other nuts

1 ½ cups cooked wholegrain rice or quinoa

1 tbsp tomato puree

- Preheat oven to 180C/350F degrees gas 5/6
- Cut off tops of the peppers and remove seeds and membrane.
- Place on a suitable baking tray
- Heat oil in a frying pan or wok; add onion and garlic, sauté 1 minute.
- Add herbs, carrots and other vegetables
- Cook 3 to 5 minutes or until carrots are tender
- Reduce heat and add the tomato, pine nuts or other nuts, rice and tomato puree

- Stuff the mixture into peppers, don't worry if it overflows
- Bake in oven for 30 minutes or until peppers feel cooked to your liking

This can have a variety of vegetables or grains so make up your own stuffing and remember you can use this to stuff any stuffable vegetable. Try making a spicy one.

THE HEALTHY TART'S SUPER SHOPPING LIST

- CHECK ALL LABELS TO ENSURE YOU ARE AVOIDING THE FOODS, ADDITIVES, INGREDIENTS THAT YOU ARE NOT SUPPOSED TO BE HAVING
- BUY ORGANIC WHERE POSSIBLE
- BUY WHAT IS IN SEASON AND LOCAL WHERE POSSIBLE

Store Cupboard Ingredient (Just a few ideas)

Rice Crackers, Oat Cakes, Corn Crackers

Porridge Oats, Millet, Quinoa *(pronounced "keen wa"),* buckwheat, Bulgur Wheat, Wholegrain rice *(basmati is good)*

Lentils, (green, red, brown) , Chick Peas, Mung beans, Black Turtle Beans, Black eyed beans, Kidney Beans, Flageolet Beans, Haricot Beans, Pinto Beans, butter beans. *(All beans may be bought in tins but check no sugar/salt, cheaper to do your own from dried, see also sprouting.*

Yeast Free Stock Marigold Swiss Boullion is good, low salt

Corn Flour, Rice Flour, Potato Flour, Soya Flour *(if you are going to do a lot of cooking/baking the different types of flour are useful)*

Rice Noodles, Rice pasta or corn pasta *(the latter minimal use)*

Herbs   *(dried are ok but fresh where possible for better flavor)*

Spices *(will be dried in powder or seeds, use seeds where possible)*

Seaweeds, Nori Wakame, Kombu, Dulse, Arame, Hijiki, Agar, Laver

Shitake and Porcini dried mushrooms

Tamari Sauce, Piri Piri, Balsamic Vinegar, Cider Vinegar, Tahini, *(check those labels!)*

Extra Virgin Olive Oil, Canola Oil, Sesame Oil, Walnut Oil, Coconut oil,

Coconut Milk, cream

Tinned Tomatoes   (ok if fresh not available, check no sugar/salt)

Sunflower, Pumpkin, Sesame, Hemp, Flax/Linseeds, *don't forget you can sprout these*

Black pepper, rock salt *(salt minimum use)*, mustard powder

Fresh Ingredients, just a few ideas, buy what is in season and of course what you fancy

Fresh chilies, ginger, garlic

Fresh vegetables/salads and fruit, carrots, swede, turnips, parsnip, kolrhabi, sweet potato, squash/pumpkin, beetroot, onions, garlic, scallions, shallots, artichokes, Cabbage red/green/white, spinach, kale, broccoli, brussel sprouts, cauliflower, asparagus. Swiss chard, Green beans. Various herb leaves, lettuce, cucumber, courgette (zucchini), peppers, celery, aubergine,

Tofu in the refrigerator department (no flesh on the 30 day plan)

Lemons and Limes *(sliced added to hot water or for salad dressings)*

Hummus, Guacamole, *(check the ingredients as you could make your own quite easily)*

It's a good idea to keep a journal of the foods you eat on a daily basis. We have provided a template that you can download off my website and print on a weekly basis to track your intake. Go to www.TrishaStewart.com and head for the download section.

DETAIL DIVAS *Fact File*

I know there are many readers who want more facts, data and details...a deeper, more technical look at some of the points I've made in this book. I also know that including it among the lists, steps and stories can feel disruptive.

That's why I've created these appendices as a resource or guide you can refer to for more information when you're ready to get the facts. After reading what is here, if you have still have questions, please contact me through the website (www.TrishaStewart.com) for more information.

Fact File A: *The BEST System Explained*

Fact File B: *Organs And What They Do*

Fact File C: *The Digestive System*

Fact File D: *The Immune System & How It Works*

Fact File E: *The Endocrine System Breakdown*

Fact File F: *Cookware: The Facts About Your Pans*

Fact File G: *Sprouting: Getting Started*

Fact File H: *Herbs: Cooking & Benefits*

Fact File I: *Food Prep & Cooking For Healthy Tarts*

Fact File J: *Vitamins & Minerals: Food Sources & Benefits*

Fact File K: *Choosing To Eat Meat*

Fact File L: *Glycaemic Index*

Fact File M: *Sugar By Any Other Name Is Still Sugar*

Fact File N: *The Truth About Artificial Sweeteners*

Fact File O: *Heavy Metals - Sources & Symptoms*

Fact File P: *How to Handle & Avoid Moldy Food*

Fact File A

The BioEnergetic Stress Testing (BEST) System
Computerized Health Screening

The Scientific Approach to Health Screening

The BEST (BioEnergetic Stress Testing) System represents the very latest in health screening technology. The System is fast, comprehensive and accurate. What is more, it is non-invasive and painless. There is no waiting around for the results – a detailed computer printout is available as soon as screening is completed, so both patient and practitioner know the situation immediately.

The BEST System has the ability to screen rapidly for reactions to chemicals, pesticides, heavy metals (such as the mercury in dental amalgams), bacteria, viruses, drugs, radiation, amino acids, vitamins, minerals, phenolics, hormones, alcohols, moulds, fungi, pollens, yeast, animal danders, toxins and more. It can screen hundreds of items for sensitivities under many categories. For example, it takes only 30 minutes to test for intolerance to 105 foods. Also screening for things like vitamin and mineral status or to establish whether dental fillings are leaking mercury into the body are easily carried out. The System can also be used to conduct more comprehensive screening of the entire body and its main organs such as the heart, lungs, liver and spleen.

Although based on acupuncture, the BEST System measures the points by pressing, as in acu*pressure*, rather than the skin penetration of acu*puncture* needles.   This is an important feature of the BEST System's non-invasive design.

Using the System, the operator applies a probe to the skin surface at the acupuncture points on the client's hands (and the feet in the case of full body screening).   The computer sends a very small electronic signal (5 volts @ 30 microamps) through the skin, via the System's negative and positive contacts.   The client only feels the sensation of the probe touching the skin.   Readings indicating the individual's reaction are recorded by the computer as each point is measured.

The natural homeostasis of energy and temperature of a healthy human is constant.   The body will always try to regulate it back to a balanced point.   Just as a thermometer is used to read temperature, a highly sensitive galvanometer is used in the BEST System to monitor variations in the energy resistance of the human body.

The body's bio System consists of acupuncture control points on the hands and feet - with 'control' or primary points on each meridian.   A balanced reading for normal (healthy) acupuncture points is 100,000 ohms.

On the BEST System the balanced reading has been set at 50 on a scale of 1 to 100.   Readings above 55 indicate an acute situation while those below 45 indicate a chronic condition. The control points indicate the overall function of say, the heart, whereas other points along the same meridian will give detailed readings – for instance, of the valves, muscles, nerves, plexus and ganglia of the heart.

A detailed report indicates the balanced, chronic and acute points relating to the various parts of the body, on both the left and right side.   The practitioner can then access the 30,000 plus remedies on the BEST System to establish the most appropriate remedy needed to rebalance the points.

The remedies are either homoeopathic or remedies evaluated using the homoeopathic approach (dilution's) from the many thousands of items loaded into the BEST System's memory. These items include bacteria, viruses, chemicals, homoeopathics (733 main items), pesticides, sensitivities, products and many more categories.   This means that the exact remedy and potency can be determined, providing dramatically improved accuracy and removing the guesswork inherent in much contemporary diagnosis.

History

In the 1950's Doctor Reinhold Voll a Germany biophysicist discovered a way to measure the energy level of bio-points (life-energy points used in Acupuncture) with an electrical devise.   Through these measurements he could:

- Screen the energy levels of the organs in the body.
- Identify toxic substances, metals, microbes, etc. that would affect the smooth functioning of the body.
- Measure food intolerance's and vitamin and mineral profile.

More importantly, he also discovered that through these same acupuncture bio-points, the effect of toxic chemicals and microbes could be minimized and corrective remedies could be identified.

The major obstacle to putting Voll's work into practice was the screening method. The technique was complicated and cumbersome which meant it was too difficult for most practitioners to use in a practical and efficient way. They had to acquire large numbers of phials, containing the substances to be screened, if they were to carry out truly comprehensive screenings.

During the last 25 years some specialized electrodermal screening developers in USA, have been perfecting a computer system that is capable of taking these measurements quickly, simply and accurately. The substances to be tested (now numbering over 30,000) were programmed into the System and a report can be generated after each screening, showing the substances tested and the results. Today, with the BEST System, instead of a few scribbled practitioner's notes, the client can receive a detailed personal report to take away and study at their leisure.

Fact File B
Organs and What They Do

Your Liver

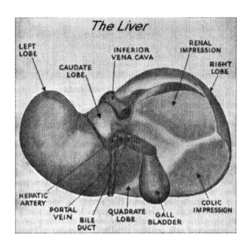

The amazing Liver is your body's own factory.   It takes deliveries, has its own sorting team and efficient distribution mechanisms.

It is the largest organ of the body and weighs in at around 3lb

There are portal veins carrying blood from the stomach, spleen, pancreas and small and large intestines so you can see why it is such an important part of digestion and immune function.

Digestive

✓ Converts glucose to glucagon so that it can store for future energy production at which point it is converted back to glucose.

✓ Metabolizes fat, it converts fat to a form in which it can be used by the tissues for energy

✓ Protein metabolism is the breakdown of amino acids which is the by product of protein if you remember from the digestive system. Removing the nitrogenous part of the amino acids which is not required to form new protein, then it is turned into urea which is then excreted in urine. It is also where new, non essential amino acids are formed, those we do not need to get from food because our liver makes them for us.

✓ Carrots and some green leaves provide us with carotene, the liver synthesizes it and give us Vitamin A as we cannot get vitamin A directly from foods.

✓ Fat Soluble vitamins A D E K are stored as well as copper and iron, unlike most of the other vitamins and minerals which are water soluble. This is why we must not overdose on ADEK because our liver may be storing them for us.

✓ Another really important link is that of the Gallbladder
  – the liver makes bile to be transported to the
  gallbladder so that it can emulsify fat.

Hormonal and Immune

✓ Regulates blood clotting

✓ Destroys erythrocytes and defends against microbes
  which means it is helping the immune system to be
  efficient

✓ Detoxifies all the noxious substances that enter our
  bodies even those we did not invite in. Chemicals in
  the food chain, fertilizers, fungicides, herbicides and
  pesticides, these could all be on non organic apples !
  as well as anywhere else in the food chain. Hormones,
  antibiotics and other drugs used in agriculture, flavors,
  colors, preservatives, solvents, chemicals in the water
  supply, alcohol and so on......plus all the pollution,
  body and hair products....the list goes on and your liver
  has to do ALL of this work, no wonder it gets hot.

✓ There are two procedures for dealing with the toxins,
  Activation which gets them out of storage and
  conjugation which means they are combined with
  other substances and eliminated as waste. If the liver
  is not efficient these toxins can be activated or let

loose and cause free radical damage which can affect the brain and mood factors. So the tidier your factory unit is the easier it can collect, re-arrange and distribute.

✓ Inactivation of hormones including insulin and glucagon, those involved in the digestive system and also those of the hormonal or endocrine system mainly the Thyroid, Cortisol (stress hormone) and the sex hormones. So here is an example of how the digestion and hormones are linked.

✓ The liver also produces heat, as it uses lots of energy performing all the jobs it has to do.

Your Kidneys

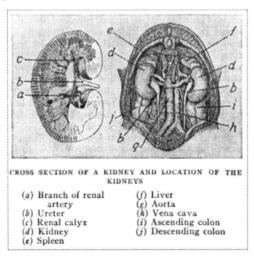

CROSS SECTION OF A KIDNEY AND LOCATION OF THE KIDNEYS

(a) Branch of renal artery
(b) Ureter
(c) Renal calyx
(d) Kidney
(e) Spleen
(f) Liver
(g) Aorta
(h) Vena cava
(i) Ascending colon
(j) Descending colon

So what have these two organs got to do with diet? Elimination of toxins, that's what.

The kidneys are sophisticated reprocessing machines. Every day your kidneys process about 180 – 200 liters of blood extracting around 2 liters of waste products and water. This becomes urine which flows to your bladder through tubes called ureters. The bladder then stores the urine until the brain sends a signal to tell you it is full and you need to empty it.

The wastes in your blood come from the normal breakdown of active tissues and from the food you eat. If your kidneys did not remove these wastes, the wastes would build up in the blood causing a toxic system.

The actual filtering occurs in tiny units inside your kidneys called nephrons. Every kidney has about a million nephrons. In the nephron, a glomerulus—which is a tiny blood vessel, or capillary—intertwines with a tiny urine-collecting tube called a tubule. A complicated chemical exchange takes place, as waste materials and water leave your blood and enter your urinary system.

You have 7 to 8 liters of blood in your body, which gets filtered approximately 20 to 25 times each day. That is a lot of filtering.

Your kidneys sift out minerals like sodium, phosphorus, and potassium and release them back to the blood to return to the body. In this way, your kidneys regulate the body's level of these substances. The right balance is necessary for health and is called homeostasis.

Your kidneys receive the blood from the **renal artery**, process it, return the processed blood to the body through the **renal vein** and remove the wastes and other unwanted substances in the urine.

If there is too much water in the body the kidneys excrete this in urine, if there is not enough due to dehydration the urine becomes more concentrated and you will notice a darker color due to the waste.

It is important to drink plenty of fresh, spring water, by the time you are thirsty you are already dehydrated.

Kidney stones, a very painful condition can be caused by too much acid in the diet and dehydration, whereby stones can be formed, they can sometimes be passed but if you can imagine one travelling down the little ureter tubes and out through your urethra! Apparently anyone who ever has one says the pain in like nothing else they have ever experienced, I guess a comparison to child birth, never had stones!!

Other kidney conditions caused by lack of water or too many toxins can be inflammation, high blood pressure, diabetic kidney, plus infections caused by toxic kidneys, just a few little reasons to ensure you cleanse and rehydrate.

Your Pancreas

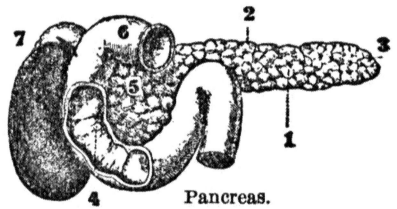

Pancreas.

1. Pancreas. 2. Body. 3. Tail. 4. Bile-duct. 5. Head.
6. Duodenum. 7. Kidney.

This is a dual gland, it is involved in the endocrine (hormonal) system and the digestive system.

Digestion

This gland produces enzymes Lipase to break down fat and Amylase to break down carbohydrates, it also produces trypsinogen and chymotrypsin to break down proteins.

Hormonally

This gland produces insulin which regulates the breaking down of carbohydrates in the system and Glucagon which increases the glucose (sugar) in the blood and Somatostatin which reduces the production of insulin and glucagon.

So here we can see how our hormones affect our digestion or the other way around.

Overuse of processed and junk food as well as highly refined sugars will all cause the pancreas to be overworked, stress is another major player here as you have seen in "fight of flight.

Type II Diabetes is now becoming an epidemic not just in adults over the age of around 50 but in children. It occurs when the pancreas fails to do its job due to overload and its then inability to either produce enough insulin or to utilize it. Type II can be controlled by diet.

Diabetes can cause blindness, kidney failure, limb amputations and heart disease. This is why your diet is so important.

Your Skin

This is the largest excretory organ, covering the whole of the outside of your body and interestingly enough the inside there is a whole layer of what we call mucous membrane covering the inside.

The skin is there to protect us from invasion by microbes such as bacteria, chemicals, pesticides etc. It contains sensory nerve endings that let us know something is hot and is also involved in the regulation of body temperature.

It contains blood vessels, sweat glands, hairs, sebaceous glands (producing oil) muscle fibers and yes, our nails, they are there to protect our fingers. And, this is where a substance is activated by the sun to produce Vitamin D.

When the body produces heat through exercise, digestion or heat generated by the liver, this make us sweat and the by products of the combustion of heat is filtered out through the sweat glands in the skin. As I have said, what comes out is what has been put in, so a clean internal environment will mean that your sweat will not smell.

Poor diet, constipation, stress causing hormonal imbalances will all affect the skin. This combination will cause spots, eczema, psoriases, rashes, dry skin, bumpy arms, acne, as well as smelly feet, armpits and so on.

We have talked about keeping the skin clean and while cleansing the internal environment it is vital to keep the external one clean as the waste coming out will be toxic.

Fact File C
The Digestive System

Let me describe your digestive system so that you will understand how it is such an important part of being full of vitality – if it is overburdened or weakened then so will you be.

The organs of digestion
- **Mouth** – containing the tongue with nerve endings of the sense of taste and teeth for chewing and salivary glands to excrete enzymes to break down the carbohydrates
- **Pharynx** – food passes from the mouth to the oesophagus
- **Oesophagus** – a long tract which propels food to the stomach
- **Stomach** – food is acted on by the acid and enzymes and is churned to a liquid chyme to be transported to the small intestine
- **Small Intestine** – The chyme is mixed with pancreatic juice, bile and intestinal juice and this is where carbohydrates are converted to monosaccharides, protein to amino acids and fats to fatty acids and glycerol and transported to the blood and lymph system for release into the body to repair, renew and build the cells
- **Large Intestine** – absorbs water, distributes mineral salts and vitamins to the blood capillaries, faeces are formed to a semi solid consistency to be transported to the rectum
- **Rectum and anal canal** – Waste leaves the body

The associated organs (those that help with digestion)
- **Salivary glands** – produce enzymes to help break down carbohydrates
- **Pancreas** – produces pancreatic juice to help digest carbohydrates, proteins and fats
- **Liver and Bile tract** – the liver produces bile which is transports to the gallbladder and the bile tract transports the bile to the stomach (duodenum)

The digestive process is that which simplifies the food you eat until they are in a form that is suitable for absorption. This is the mechanical breakdown of foods by chewing and the chemical breakdown of food by the enzymes present in secretions produced by the glands and accessory organs.

Absorption is the process by which the digested foods pass through the walls of the organs of the digestive system into the blood and lymph capillaries for circulation around the body.

Elimination is when the food that cannot be digested (fiber) is excreted by the bowel.

There are of course many other complicated systems and organs of the body which play a very important part in the digestive system including hormones, kidneys, liver, pancreas, spleen and so on – you can learn more about these by reading the other Fact Files in this book or go to www.trishastewart.com for a more comprehensive look.

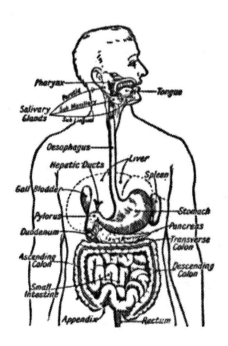

Fact File D
The Immune System and Your Defenses

The body consists of a lymphatic system, which is not unlike the vascular or blood system as it has fluid flowing through capillaries; the fluids, however, are not blood but clear lymphatic fluids. Unlike the blood system where the heart pumps the blood around the body, lymphatic fluids rely on muscular contraction to pump the fluid through the capillaries and around the body through a series of nodes, glands or vessels including the spleen which contains cells to destroy foreign invaders. This is one reason why exercise is so important.

The main nodes are situated in the neck, armpits, abdomen and groin. You may have noticed swelling in any of these areas when you have had an infection; this is because they are working hard to destroy bacteria, viruses and other foreign invaders.

The following are also involved in immunity or protection

- The skin outside the body and other lining tissues inside forming a barrier
- Mucus lining of the gut and lungs which traps invading bacteria
- Hairs which move the mucus and trapped bacteria out of the lungs
- Stomach acid which kills bacteria that have been swallowed
- Helpful bacteria growing in the bowel which prevent other bacteria from taking over

- Urine flow which flushes bacteria out of the bladder and urethra
- White blood cells called 'neutrophils' which can find and kill bacteria and other infectious agents

So, what are these cells and where are they produced?

Bone Marrow
Generates specialized cells, some of which mature into B cells while others travel into the circulation and to the Thymus where they mature into T cells.

What do B cells do?
They produce antibodies which target specific foreign invaders (or antigens). The antibody made is different for each invader or antigen. The antibody clings onto the surface of the invading bacteria or virus. The invader is then marked with the antibody so that the body knows it is dangerous and it can be killed off. The next time this bacteria or virus tries to invade the B cells, which have a memory, they will be ready to zap it very quickly. This is building your immunity step by step because every time a foreign invader invites itself in, these cells will produce another antibody to protect you.

What do T cells do?
They are trained to differentiate between invader and friend so they are "helpers" and "killers". The helpers stimulate the B cells to make antibodies and help to develop the "killer" T cells which then go on to "kill" the cells that have been invaded by the foreign invaders; which could be bacteria or viruses.

What about the white blood cells that are always talked about. Where are they and what do they do?

These cells are called leukocytes and are made up of other cells. They travel in the vascular or blood system and are very important for fighting infection. They are good at fighting bacterial and fungal infections.

They can move to sites of infection in the body including burns and wounds, stick to invading bacteria or fungi, swallow up the invader which they then carry off to the lymph nodes for destruction.

We are told as children that the more bacteria and viruses we are up against the better our immunity will work! Well that is all well and good but what about when it doesn't work, when the body immunity breaks down. Let's go for my "totting up" system here again and say that the following will invade our immunity:

- Junk Food and all those BAD and UGLY foods we have mentioned because eventually your digestive system, which contains lots of lymphoid tissue, will break down (see digestive system in appendices) and cause what we term "leaky gut syndrome" where this tissue has broken down and allows partially digested foods into the blood system.

   This will look like foreign invaders and the immune system will want to zap them. Continually doing this will weaken the immune system or at the least it will be kept too busy (through being overworked) to properly protect other areas

- Toxins ingested into the body either by pollution or those body sprays, toothpaste and all those things we have mentioned in the 'Good, Bad and Very Ugly' will eventually overtax the immune system and much more.

- Stress will weaken us and can cause a systemic overload which will affect our immunity

Is it any wonder that we are seeing so many cases nowadays of chronic fatigue, fibromyalgia and various cancers? When the immune system gets so weakened and compromised, it can no longer fight off these ailments and diseases.

And of course we must remember those autoimmune diseases such as rheumatoid arthritis, multiple sclerosis, lupus, Hasimoto's and Graves disease (under and over active thyroid/thyroiditis); where the body attacks itself and has lost control over its own defenses.

Our personal Eden has good wholesome organic food, clean water, is chemical free, preservative free, and protects us from all that 'modern day' junk that compromises our immune systems.

Whenever you put something in your mouth, there are consequences for every organ in your body. So STOP putting junk into your body. Your organs will thank you, your immune system will thank you and you'll look better and stay healthier!

Fact File E
The Endocrine System Breakdown

The adrenal system

The adrenal hormones which are made up of adrenaline (epinephrine) and noradrenalin (norepinephrine)... are triggered as a response to physical or mental stress. Cortisol (hydrocortisone), one of the glucocorticoids, raises the blood sugar (glucose) by stimulating gluconeogenesis in the liver which converts that stored fat and protein into glucose so that the body can use it. Cortisol also has an anti-inflammatory response.

The adrenal, or suprarenal, gland is paired with one gland located near the upper portion of each kidney. Each gland is divided into an outer cortex and an inner medulla. The cortex and medulla of the adrenal gland, like the anterior and posterior lobes of the pituitary, develop from different embryonic tissues and secrete different hormones. The adrenal cortex is essential to life, but the medulla may be removed with no life-threatening effects.

The hypothalamus of the brain influences both portions of the adrenal gland but by different mechanisms. The adrenal cortex is regulated by negative feedback involving the hypothalamus and adrenocorticotropic hormone; the medulla is regulated by nerve impulses from the hypothalamus.

Hormones of the Adrenal Cortex

The adrenal cortex consists of three different regions, with each region producing a different group or type of hormones. Chemically, all the cortical hormones are steroid. Mineralocorticoids are secreted by the outermost region of the adrenal cortex. The principal mineralocorticoid is aldosterone, which acts to conserve sodium ions and water in the body. Glucocorticoids are secreted by the middle region of the adrenal cortex. The principal glucocorticoid is cortisol, which increases blood glucose levels. The third group of steroids secreted by the adrenal cortex is the gonadocorticoids, or sex hormones. These are secreted by the innermost region. Male hormones (androgens) and female hormones (estrogens) are secreted in minimal amounts in both sexes by the adrenal cortex, but their effect is usually masked by the hormones from the testes and ovaries. In females, the masculinization effect of androgen secretion may become evident after menopause, when estrogen levels from the ovaries decrease.

Hormones of the Adrenal Medulla

The adrenal medulla develops from neural tissue and secretes two hormones, epinephrine and norepinephrine. These two hormones are secreted in response to stimulation by sympathetic nerves, particularly during stressful situations. A lack of hormones from the adrenal medulla produces no significant effects. Hyper secretion, usually from a tumor, causes prolonged or continual sympathetic responses.

Over two dozen hormones and chemicals have been identified in various parts of the gastrointestinal system. Here are a few that will help you to understand how they affect digestion:

Cholecystokinin (CCK) - It is secreted by cells in the duodenum and jejunum (parts of the stomach) when they are exposed to food. It acts on the gall bladder stimulating it to contract and force its contents of bile into the intestine and stimulates the pancreas into the release of digestive enzymes into the pancreatic fluid. CCK also acts on vagal neurons (nerve) leading back to the medulla oblongata (brain stem) which give a signal to let you know you have eaten enough...how many ignore that one!!! This is an interesting subject as the Vagus Nerve is attached to the brain stem, its path is down the esophagus and breaks into the stomach...hence "butterflies" or IBS is caused by stress...it's that "sick to my stomach feeling" you can get when you're nervous or anxious.

Gastrin: Is secreted by the cells in the stomach and duodenum, thus encouraging stomach acid (hydrochloric acid) and pepsin.

Secretin: Is secreted by the duodenum, it calls upon the pancreas to produce bicarbonate to suppress the acidity of the stomach. Imagine the work all this lot has to do when you eat or drink a mix of too many spicy or acidic foods and liquids!!

GIP (Gastric Inhibitory Peptide)

Food in the duodenum stimulates certain endocrine cells to produce GIP. This has the opposite effects of gastrin; it inhibits gastric glands in the stomach and it inhibits the mixing and churning movement of stomach muscles. This slows the rate of stomach emptying when the duodenum contains food.

Fact File F

Cookware: The Facts about Your Pans

Aluminum

The perils of aluminum pans have been well known for sometime and as you will have read in Chapter six there is already far too much of this metal in the food chain and in body products. Aluminum has been associated with Alzheimer's disease but there is no definite proof as yet. The World Health Organization estimates that adults can consume more than 50 milligrams of aluminum daily without harm, no thanks is what I say.

As with any metal cookware there will be a certain amount that will leach into foods, particularly those foods such as leafy vegetables, citrus and tomatoes. The problem with aluminum is that it dissolves most easily from worn or pitted pots and pans.

Anodized Aluminum Cookware

There is a slight improvement using this type of cookware as the surface is harder and non scratch therefore reducing the amount or the possibility of leaching into foods.

Copper

The cookware of the professionals as the heat is evenly distributed. Copper in small amounts is good for us but like anything a large amount can be toxic and also coming from a pan, what else may be in this? Copper pans often come with a stainless steel cooking surface so these could be used.

Stainless Steel and Iron Cookware

Stainless steel and Iron cookware are probably the safest depending on any other metal that is mixed with it during the manufacturing process.

Nickel and Chromium are probably the two metals that may leach out of this cookware in small quantities and relatively harmless but remember the "totting up" system I use and the fact that all these metals are in packaged/processed foods, body and hair products and cleaning materials.

Ceramic

Ceramic cookware is glazed; similar glazes are applied to metals to make enamelware. These glazes, a form of glass, resist wear and corrosion.

The problem here is the use of pigments such as lead and cadmium in making the glaze and the chemicals involved.

Glass

This material should be harmless unless of course there are chemicals that go into the glazing. The problem is heating to high temperatures.

Plastics

For cooking and storing food are fine as long as there is not heat placed upon them, so using in a microwave could prove to be harmful. Using plastic containers and wrap for anything other than their original purpose may cause health problems. Wrapping foods in plastic cling film again is ok but do not add heat because this will release chemicals that can harm us. Plastic is known to be estrogenic and therefore may be linked to infertility in men.

Non-stick

There has been lots of news on non-stick coatings which are applied to metal pans to prevent food from sticking and help reduce the amount of oil needed. The coating is likely to be carcinogenic, there are several independent studies performed on rats which of course like all these studies is appalling. The product widely used in the coating is Perfluorootanoic and its salts known as PFOA. The biggest problem is the poisonous fumes from the coating when the pans are heated.

So what can you do? You have to cook or store foods!
Minimize your risks by the following:

- It would be a good idea to get rid of all aluminum cookware, if you decide not to, do not store cooked foods in these pans.

- As we said in Step Two get rid of all cookware that is chipped, flaking or not at its best.
- Beware of nickel if you are allergic or have an intolerance to it
- Do not store any citrus fruits, green leafy vegetables or tomato based meals in any metal pan
- Do not heat plastic bowls or cling film
- If using ceramic beware of cheap products as they may contain chemicals in the manufacture and glazing.

Fact File G
Sprouting: Getting Started

So, how do you get started? It's really quite simple...just select the seeds you'd like to sprout (I've provided a partial list below). Then follow these easy steps:

- Get your container cleaned and ready
- Soak the seeds or whatever you are going to sprout overnight
- Drain and rinse in the morning
- Place in the container you are going to grow them in, this could be a jar, colander, basket, hemp sprout bag or seed tray
- Rinse again, preferably with a spray attachment.
- Rinse twice a day...once in the morning and once at night

Harvest!! You're ready when the seeds are sprouting leaves or shoots. The actual growing time will vary depending on the seeds or beans.

Fact File H
Herbs: Cooking & Benefits

Bay Leaf (sweet laurel): This spicy, aromatic herb is used in cooking for soups, casseroles, bouquet garni, meat and fish dishes. But, what makes it even more worthwhile is its qualities that aid digestion, reduce flatulence and it's known to treat influenza and bronchitis. Also, an infusion of the crushed berries acts like a diuretic and is anti-rheumatic. Fresh is milder than dried but both are excellent in cooking.

Basil (sweet): The Italian ingredient for pesto...the French dash for Provencal soupe au pisto...with its wonderful aroma, fresh is definitely best here. It's ideal with tomatoes, tomato soup, salad, eggs and more. Therapeutic uses for basil include use as a sedative and anti-spasmodic; it's also helpful with digestion, nervous disorders, headaches, vertigo and even colic in children. It's also been said that the fresh juice from the leaves poured into the ears will ease inflammation and an infusion makes a great gargle for thrush.

Dill: Although mainly used for cooking with fish (by the way...it's best raw) or in making things like dill pickles. Also, dill soaked overnight in water makes a mild 'tea' that helps to calm the stomach.

Marjoram: This beauty blends well with Thyme and Basil for sauces, vegetable casseroles and the like. Medicinally, it's a sedative (small does only), soothes the digestive system and helps with the endocrine (hormonal) system. Its antiseptic values are used for tonsillitis, colds and respiratory problems. Plus, it's used in compresses and lotions to aid wound healing and is known for its relaxation and calming effects.

Mint: Perhaps one of the better know herbs...it comes in several varieties. For food uses, it makes everything from a great tea to jelly to sauce. Its 'non-food' qualities make it ideal for antiseptics, mouth wash and even digestive aids.

Parsley: Oh you know this one...that garnish everyone leaves on their plate!!! Well, leave it no more...eat it. That's right it's perfect to combat the smell of garlic on your breath! Parsley juice is a good mosquito repellent, mild laxative and diuretic. It's mild but fulfilling flavor is why it's used in so many recipes...plus it's rich in Vitamin C, iron, magnesium and other vitamins and minerals. Parsley...it's more than plate decoration!

Rosemary: Almost synonymous with lamb, its culinary uses are mainly for meats, stews and soups. But this great smelling herb is a stimulant and rosemary tonics can be beneficial for invalids and depressives. Did you know it symbolizes love, friendship and fidelity? Pick up a plant today...the trailing variety is beautiful and hardy.

Sage: Sage has many varieties, but they're all lovely with a number of dishes including stews, casseroles and roasted vegetables. Its distinctive flavor is a must in many households when making 'dressing' or 'stuffing'. Sage also has medicinal values for treating PMS and menopause, soothing pain, as a nervous system regulator and helps stimulate circulation.

Tarragon: It's a common staple in many cooking sauces, marinades and stuffing. Medicinally it is often used to aid healthy digestion.

Thyme: Let's just get straight to the therapeutic benefits...it makes a good tonic to help with digestion, circulation, coughs, colds and regulating hormones. In the kitchen, it's similar to rosemary in that it's used a great deal in bouquet garni, for soups, stews, casseroles and vegetable dishes.

Coriander (green plant): Although many herbs are similar in flavor and use whether dried or fresh...that's not so with coriander. The flavor of the fresh leaf is quite different from the seeds. Primarily used in salads and curries, if you're working with the fresh leaf...use it toward the end of the cooking, but with seeds...use at the beginning. Its medicinal purposes are thought to help eliminate toxic waste such as

metals from the body including mercury...tooth fillings...,
cadmium and lead.

Whew! There are many more herbs I could talk about, but
these are the basics you probably already have in some form
in your kitchen. You can easily see how vital herbs are to a
Healthy Tart lifestyle. Not only in the kitchen to jazz up
meals, but to support good health...especially good digestion.
They help to produce enzymes and are enriched with vitamins
and minerals. Check out www.TrishaStewart.com for more
details on cooking and healing with herbs.

Fact File I

Food Prep & Cooking For Healthy Tarts

Here are some food prep and cooking tips to get even the most novice of cooks on the road to being a Healthy Tart. Many of you may know this information, but refreshers are always good. And, you may find a few tips and ideas that will help you make your cooking easier and more nutritious!

The following two types of rice are those I would recommend for your immediate work towards becoming a Healthy Tart, others will be explained in the cookery book or on the website

1. Wholegrain Basmati rice is one of my favorites. It takes longer to cook, is far more nutritious than white or other rice as it has a slower release of energy to keep you going. It has the outer husk removed whilst the bran a germ are intact. Use twice the amount of water to rice, bring to the boil and simmer with the lid on until most of the water is absorbed.

2. Wild Rice is actually an aquatic grass, it is a dramatic brown/black color and is nutty, takes longer than most grains to cook but can be soaked overnight to reduce the time. It is very nutritious as it contains all the essential amino acids and is rich in lysine and is also gluten free. Cook as above

Other rice includes white long grain which most people choose, of no nutrient value, short grain or pudding rice, Jasmine, Red Carmargue, Aborio for risottos, Valencia for Paella, Japanese Sushi rice

Rice flour is a great alternative to wheat flour as it is gluten free

Rice pasta is also a great alternative to wheat pasta.

How to keep rice or other grain

- Keep a batch over no more than 3 days
- Cook according to which grain you are using and rinse off with cold water, drain and put in the fridge except for the portion you may be using at that meal. This will ensure that when you want to throw a grain dish together you already have the base ingredients.
- Should you wish to refresh and use hot, bring a pan of water to the boil, put the grain in and bring back to the boil for 60 seconds
- You can also sauté the grain if making a risotto the fast way
- Cold is always ready for your salad

The benefits of eating wholegrains and whole cereals include a slow release of carbohydrate (low GI or GL) low fat, good source of protein, fiber, vitamins and minerals,

Other Grains or cereals that we will use during the 30 day plan and of course beyond

- Oats come in jumbo, rolled, flaked, oatmeal, oat bran for making porridge and oatcakes plus many other uses. Whole oats have the germ and the bran intact anything less than whole will give less benefits. These are glutinous and should be avoided by people with a gluten intolerance or celiac disease.
- Quinoia (Pronounced keen-wah) is a super grain as it contains all the essential amino acids and is gluten free. Does not take as long as wholegrain rice to cook but does double in size. As a rule of thumb for one person ½ cup quinoa to 1 cup of water, bring to boil and simmer with the lid on.

- Millet grains, flakes and flour are gluten free. Ideal for porridge or use as a change from rice.
- Buckwheat is not wheat but of the Rhubarb family. Gluten free, comes plain or toasted and is used in pancakes from the buckwheat flour, porridge (Kasha) and Japanese soba noodles.
- Barley, most people know this as pearl or pot barley. Pot barley is more nutritious as it is the wholegrain. Great in soups and casseroles. Barley flakes can be used for porridge or muesli making.

Others such as wheat, wheat berries, cracked wheat, wheat germ, flakes, wheat bran, seitan, rye, corn, cornmeal, cornflour, amaranth, sorghum, spelt, kamut, will be further explained in the cookery book or website.

Legumes very versatile and nutritious food with a range of shapes and textures. They are an important part of protein in a vegetarian diet as well as fiber, vitamins and minerals. They are low in fat, low GI/GL so slow release of carbohydrates.

- Red, yellow, green, brown, puy are all lentils. These do not need soaking, wash and pick over as there maybe stones in them. Red, split lentils have the shortest cooking time and develop into a mush and are very suited to making Dhal, as are the yellow ones. Green and brown take longer to cook and retain their shape so are ideal as they can be used for salads, casseroles etc. Puy lentils keep their shape and also look very nice, are superior in taste and texture.
- Peas, split, marrow fat are great for adding to soups and casseroles or making "mushy peas" or pease pudding. They need soaking overnight.

Pulses

These are an important part of any diet as they are packed with protein and fiber, vitamins and minerals, and extremely low in fat, low GI/GL.

Ideal fill up foods when you are on a weight-loss program. These do need to be soaked overnight. You can buy them in cans but you must choose salt and sugar free.

These can also be sprouted, see sprouting section in book.

Soak overnight or at least 5-6 hours, remove from the water and rinse, place in a large pan with water and bring to the boil, skim and simmer for 1-2 hours depending on type of bean, check for tenderness.

Do not add salt to the water as this will make them tough but to prevent flatulence add ginger, dill and caraway to the cooking water.

Some of the beans to use, all have an interesting taste and texture, choose your favorites as they will all be useful to your diet.

Aduki (adzuki), black-eyed, black turtle are often used in oriental cooking, Creole and Indian cooking, but can be used whenever you need beans.

Cannellini, Borlotti, Butter, Haricot, Flageolet, Pinto are what I would term as the softer bean, used in European cooking. Chick peas or Garbanzo are like little nuts with a creamy flavor.

Kidney well remembered for their use in South American cooking, these keep their shape and look great in salads. They do, however need special care when bringing to the boil. Boil vigorously for 10-15 minutes as they contain a substance that can cause severe food poisoning. They also require a longer soaking period of about 8-12 hours.

All of the beans will be a great addition to curry, salads, soups, casseroles, refried, mashed into a puree. Add full flavors to enhance the taste of pulses.

Soya Bean Products
Tofu or bean curd is exactly what is says, the curd from the milk of the bean. It comes in various textures, shapes and flavors. This product is high in protein, very low in fat and an excellent alternative to meat.

- Firm Tofu is in a block which can be cubed, sliced and used as kebabs, in salads, stir fry, casserole or mashed and made into burgers, rissoles, patties. This product is very bland and does improve with marinating or you can buy smoked, herbed or deep fried.

- Silken Tofu has a smoother texture and is ideal for sauces, dips, dressings. A very useful dairy alternative.

Keep covered in water and in the fridge for up to one week.

Tempeh

This is made by fermenting cooked soya beans. It is of a nuttier taste and if you are missing meat the texture is firmer and it works well in casseroles and pies.

TVP (textured vegetable protein)

Has been used for years as a meat replacement. You can buy it in mince or chunks and it has to be re-hydrated before use.

Soya flour is gluten free so a good alternative to wheat.

Soy Sauce

Is made by combining crushed soya beans, wheat, salt, water and a yeast based culture called Koji and left to ferment from 6months to 3 years. Hence you will pay more for the best quality. Try to buy naturally brewed as there are a lot of chemically prepared products on the market so they ferment faster. The dark sauce is heavier and sweeter whilst the light is thinner and saltier.

Shoyu

As above but aged for 1-2 years, has a rich, full flavor

Tamari

This product is made without the wheat so is gluten free. Can be used in cooking or as a condiment

Miso

Made from cooked soya beans, rice, wheat or barley, salt and water and is left to ferment for about 3 years. You can add it to soups, stock, stir fry and noodle dishes. There are three types, Kome or white miso is the lightest in strength, Mugi is a medium strength and Hacho is dark, rich and thick and has a strong flavor.

All of the above sauces are very salty so use sparingly.

Soya milk, cream and yoghurt are good dairy alternatives. As are rice and nut milks, creams and butters.

Nuts

Pecan, pine, walnuts, pistachio, macadamia, cashew, almonds, brazils, coconuts, (brazils and coconuts are high in saturated fat so take it easy), chestnuts, hazelnuts. Always buy as fresh as possible and in small quantities, if buying in shell they should feel heavy for their size, this will indicate freshness.

You can make nut butters by putting ½ cup shelled nuts into a food processor or blender and process until finely ground, add 1-2 tbsp of sunflower or olive oil and process to a smooth paste. Keep in the fridge.

Most nuts are high in either mono/poly unsaturated fats. Packed with protein, vitamins and minerals.

Seeds

Sesame, Sunflower, Poppy, Pumpkin, Hemp, Linseeds (flax) all rich with essential fatty acids and protein, vitamins and minerals. You can make seed butter in the same way as nut butter. Purchase in small quantities, dry roasting brings out the flavor, grinding releases the oils and is the best method for using these nutritious foods. Packed with essential fatty acids, protein, vitamins and minerals

Fruit and Vegetable Kingdom

Providing energy, fiber, vitamins and minerals, antioxidants, betacarotene, phytochemicals, Bioflavanoids, fabulous health giving properties, see the chart for details of this.

I have not listed every fruit and vegetable this will come later in the cookbook and on the website.

Roots and Tubers

Root vegetables are comforting and nourishing and popular in winter, leave the outer skins on where possible as this is a great source of natural fiber.

Carrots

These are not just a good winter vegetable as we get the summer crops also. Choose the smaller ones as they will be sweeter. Suitable to eat raw, juiced, steamed, stir fried, roasted.

Beetroot

Beetroot can have an "earthy" taste particularly when juiced. They add a fabulous color to salads if grated, used in risottos or soups or roasted, mashed. Take care when washing so the skin does not get damaged as the red color will leach out. Choose firm products do not accept them if the skin is wrinkly they will be old and woody. Beetroot has always been considered a "tonic" to help disorders of the blood including anaemia.

Celeriac

Similar in flavor to celery. This must be peeled but can be eaten raw, cooked and mashed, baked, steamed or in a soup. Try mashing with other roots to get a blend of flavors. Great topping for vegetable bakes.

Parsnip

Sweet and works well roasted, mashed, pureed, grated or I love them with carrots in a risotto These are best bought after the first frost as it is said the cold converts the starch into sugar enhancing its sweetness. Avoid old or limp products as they will be woody and not at all nice.

Swede

Good raw, steamed, mashed and as a mix with others that mash.

Turnips

These have a slight peppery taste, depending on their size, choose small firm ones. Boil, steam, bake, roast or raw..

Potatoes

Far too many to name, all with their distinctive flavor and uses. Do not use potatoes that have green patches. Depending on type choose your favorite way of cooking them.

Sweet Potatoes or Yams

Suited to mashing, roasting, jackets, slighter slower release of energy than the white potato.

Jerusalem Artichokes

These are often knobbly and small and a nuisance to prepare but do add a pungent flavor to soups or use as potatoes and maybe mash with others. They usually need to have the outer skin taken off.

Horseradish

Often overlooked as most people buy it in the jar. It has a pungent taste and is usually grated and mixed with cream or vinegar, try cider vinegar but can be grated into mash, sauces or soups. Opens the sinus canals !

Brassicas and Green Leafy Vegetables

Buying and Storing. These do not keep well so always buy fresh and use as soon as possible.

I find a lot of people have been put off eating some of the following vegetables because they had to eat them at school when they were boiled to death and stank ! the best way to overcome this is to shred and eat them raw a completely different flavor and far more nutritious.

Broccoli

Purple sprouting and green. Does not deserve to be boiled! Best steamed or raw. Trim the larger stalk and add into soups. Trim the florets and sprinkle raw onto salads, the kids won't even notice it !

Cauliflower

Does not deserve to be boiled, steam or eat raw, great in salads or I actually like them in my vegetable curry after they have absorbed the flavor, gives a different texture to the dish.

Cabbage

Quite a few varieties of cabbage. Try shredded and eaten raw or lightly steamed, mix with red cabbage for a colorful salad or stir fry.

Brussel Sprouts

Best after the first frost. The same as for cabbage.

Kale

This can be a little bitter if old so buy only young leaves and steam or stir fry or juice.

Spinach

A fabulous green, full of all the nutrients. Buy baby leaf and eat raw, never cook this it is too precious. The darker more mature greens only need a little light cooking, wash and let the leaves stay wet, put a pan on the heat and put in the spinach, put the lid on for a few minutes and hey presto a lovely dark green vegetable dish. Spinach apparently, does not contain the iron that "Popeye" thought it did as spinach contains oxalic acid which inhibits the absorption of iron and calcium but a fantastic cancer-fighting antioxidant with about four times more beta carotene than broccoli. So well worth eating. If you have experienced a "bitter" taste it will be due to the kind of cooking or the spinach is too old. If large leaves and not so young, take the leaves away from any thick stems and put the stems into a vegetable stock of soup.

Swiss Chard

This is a member of the beet family, used in the same way as spinach and again does contain oxalic acid.

Spring Greens

A leafy cabbage really, full flavor and yes, springtime is the best time to have this vegetable, all new, green and lush. Shred and eat raw or lightly steamed.

Pumpkins and the Squash Family

These arrive at different times of the year so there will always be a season for these versatile vegetables.

Winter Squash tends to have a tough inedible skin with a dense and fibrous flesh and large seeds and can be used in both sweet and savory dishes. These are Acorn, Butternut and Pumpkin.

Summer Squash are picked whilst young and the skins are tender, Pattypan, Courgette, Marrows and Cucumber.

Always buy fresh but Winter Squash will keep for several weeks if stored in a cool place.

When peeling the winter squash take care as the outer skins are tough. Cut into chunks that you can deal with, discard the skin and seeds although you can roast the pumpkin seeds if you like after they have been dried.

Shoot Vegetables
Fennel

Florence fennel is closely related to the herb and spice of the same name. It has a similar texture to celery. The whole vegetable including the fronds are edible. It has quite a distinct aniseed flavor but cooking encourages a sweetness. This vegetable can be sliced, chopped and included in salads, cut into quarters or eights, brushed with olive oil and roasted.

Asparagus

In the UK the season for this wonderful vegetable is late April till June although worldwide it is available at any time. A very therapeutic and visual vegetable simply cooked by poaching or roasted which almost seems a shame but gives a different dimension. Drizzle with a little olive oil.

Chicory

These are used in salads but need to be combined with sweeter leaves as they can be slightly bitter in taste. You can steam or add to a stir fry.

Celery

A very medicinal vegetable, tangy in taste, if bitter the celery is old. Eaten raw or braised but can be added to soups or included in a vegetable stock.

Vegetable Fruits
Tomatoes

An all time favorite and very versatile fruit. Vine ripened in natural sunlight so are best eaten seasonally. There are many varieties including cherry and plum. Sundried are so tasty, added to salads, stir fry, a mezze and so on, and are available all year round.

Aubergine

Little understood and an undervalued fruit. Most of us know it as being oval and deep in color. The smaller egg shaped variety is the one that has the name "eggplant" associated with it. It is a great addition to spicy casseroles, tomato based dishes such as ratatouille, Greek dishes such as Moussaka (healthy vegetarian one of course!) roasted, stuffed and pureed into dips with lots of garlic. Don't buy huge ones as they will be tough and have more seeds. Do not buy them with damaged or wrinkly skins. They absorb a lot of oil so it is advisable not to fry them.

Chilies

A member of the Capsicum family. Widely used in Indian, Mexican and other spicy dishes. Unfortunately most people use the dried powder which is ok but not quite like the fresh ones. There are many varieties and shapes ranging in potency from very mild to very hot. The smaller ones tend to be the hottest, not by color. They can be red, green, yellow or orange depending on how they have ripened in the sun. Take care when preparing, I use rubber gloves to slice open and remove the seeds and white membrane as this is where the "hot" is at its most potent. Do not touch your face or eyes as they will sting like mad.

Peppers

The same as for chilies, they come in a range of colors, the green ones are commonly less ripened which sometime makes them harder to digest although they are so tasty and crisp. The other colors are generally sweeter. Great roasted, stuffed, raw, steamed lightly and then marinated in a flavored olive oil. Great addition to all tomato based recipes.

Avocado

Not understood as a health giving fruit because it is high in fat, but the fat is monosaturated and therefore helps to lower cholesterol. Lots of protein and essential fatty acids makes this a very desirable food product. Slice in half and remove the stone, eat as it is or add a dressing or spoon in a tasty dip or cube into salads. Guacamole is a favorite dip which is mashed avocado, lemon juice, chopped sweet chillis and peppers, or anything you want.

Pods and Seeds
Peas

A great favorite for both flavor and color. Pick as young and fresh as possible as they become starchy if left too long. Can be used in any way liked, raw or cooked.

Broad Beans

Again, young and fresh are best. If they are larger you need to remove them from their pods, a fiddly job but well worth it. If they have gone "over" a little the shells can be removed after cooking.

Green Beans

We have quite a variety of these, French, Runner, Dwarf and so on. Top and tail and steam or eat raw, great with pulses and eaten with salads.

Sweet Corn

Eat soon after picking, like peas they can be a bit starchy if left and the kernels get tough. Baby corn can be eaten whole, the larger variety need to have the outer leaves removed.

The Onion Family
Onions

There are a great variety of these and used in so many ways. They range in taste from sweet and juicy to a powerful and pungent taste. Shallots are delicious roasted with garlic. Many culinary uses for onions both raw and cooked.

Garlic

Great health benefits being anti-viral and anti-fungal. Whole garlic is sweet and great roasted or cooked in many dishes. Mincing, dicing or crushing the garlic gives off a more pungent taste. Only buy garlic bulbs if they are juicy and moist. They are semi-dried which prolongs the shelf life but discard if they have green shoots coming out or are very dry. Summer or "wet" garlic looks a bit like a large spring onion and can be used in the same way as the dryer variety. Do not store in the fridge but keep in a cool dark place.

Leeks

Very versatile with a great taste, steam, sauté, add to soup or shred and stir fry. They are easy to clean, cut off the base and remove a layer of the outer skin, chop off the toughest of the green part whilst retaining some and then slice halfway through lengthways and was. These often are gritty and this will wash them all the way through.

Mushrooms

There are many books on mushroom varieties, edible or non edible, Chinese to Portobello, dried to fresh. It is well worth getting a book if you are interested in the benefits of these versatile food items. If you have an issue such as candida or a respiratory problem I do not recommend eating them as they are Fungi, grow in the damp and wet and throw off spores. See more on candida or respiratory problems at www.TrishaStewart.com

Salad Leaves

Red, dark green, light green, purple, peppery, sweet, bitter and so on. Such a variety these days which really jazz up the simplest salad or garnish. It is good to eat a raw salad with a cooked meal or as a starter as this encourages the digestive enzymes to flow.

Fruits

The ultimate convenience food, washed and eaten on the go, juiced or used in a variety of salads and bakes. Always buy firm fruits with no bruising or broken skins. They release fructose which is a natural sugar for energy. Use homegrown in season as naturally ripened fruits give off the best enzymes, vitamins and minerals, bioflavanoids and anti-oxidants. Great for digestion, kidneys, skin, hair and much more.

Apples

Several varieties from Cox's Orange Pippin to the tart flavor of a Bramley. Used in both savory and sweet dishes.

Pears

Versatile in savory and sweet dishes. Many varieties.

Apricots

So much nicer fresh than dried, raw is best, cooked gives a different flavor.

Cherries

Sweet ones are best eaten raw, Morello are sour and need cooking.

Plums

Ranging in color from pale yellow to rich purple. Many varieties sweet and tart. Can be cooked and pureed to make a sauce or fresh in a fruit combo.

Peaches and Nectarines

Very seasonal if you want them at their best. Eat raw with skin on preferably

Citrus
Oranges, lemons, limes, grapefruits

These fruits need to be eaten when they are ripened in the sunlight and not stored in some container until shipped to wherever and then ripened in storage. The benefits and versatility of these fruits are worth waiting for and getting the best from. They are great sliced in hot water to drink, grated rind in dishes, dressings, sauces or just whole fruit juiced and so on.

Berries and currants

VERY seasonal, but a great treat especially if you can pick from the hedgerows or homegrown pickings. Strawberries, Raspberries, Blackberries, Blueberries, Gooseberries,

Blackcurrants, Redcurrants, White currants, great fresh picked, juiced, pureed delightful!

Grapes, Melons, Dates and Figs

Many varieties of Grapes used in wine making, juicing and eaten whole. Melons have a high water content so great in the summer for quenching the thirst. Eat aside from any other food as they digest very quickly and can inhibit the absorption and nutrients from other foods.

Figs, such a delight when they are fresh, can be poached or baked. Dates eaten fresh are sweet and soft.

Tropical Fruit

Pineapple and Papaya are great for the digestion as they contain the enzymes bromelain and papain. Great for juicing and fruit combos. Bananas very starchy which is why they are so popular as they fill the hunger gap, mashed or blended makes a thick smoothie. Mango, check the skin for ripeness a totally green skin is the sign of an unripe fruit. Depends where you live in the world as to the seasonal availability.

Oils

These provide us with essential fatty acids, vitamins and minerals. There are a wide variety of oils for cooking and for use in dressings. They are made from fruits, nuts, seeds and best extracted by slow mechanical means rather than being put through a heat process which changes the properties. Choose first cold pressed, un-refined oils for flavor and nutrient value.

Olive Oil

Olive oil, is as it states from olives usually grown in France, Greece, Italy or Spain. Generally the hotter the climate the more robust the oil. It comes in Extra Virgin which is a premium oil and best used for dressings or just drizzled over steamed vegetables, stirred into sauces etc. Virgin is also a premium oil and is best used in the same way or mixed with lighter oils for cooking. Pure olive oil will be blended and refined, lighter in flavor and suitable for cooking.

Corn oil

Suitable for cooking.

Safflower

Light all purpose oil, contains more polyunsaturated fat than any other type of oil, made from the seeds of the safflower.

Sunflower Oil

Made from the seeds of the sunflower, good all purpose oil, not very strong in flavor. Good if mixed with olive or other oils for better flavor.

Soya oil

Useful for frying as it has a high smoking point and remains stable at high temperatures. Choose from non GM products.

Groundnut

Also know as peanut oil. Not much flavor.

Rapeseed

Bland tasting all purpose. High in monosaturated fat

Grapeseed

Delicate flavor, made from seeds of the grapes left over from winemaking. Good all round use.

Sesame

The dark variety has a nutty aroma, used for flavoring marinades and in stir fry as it has a high smoking point. Very strong in taste. The pale variety is from untoasted seeds and lighter in flavor.

Walnut

Intensely flavored and delicious in salad dressings, do not heat or cook as it is very expensive and far too good.

Hazelnut

Fine and fragrant, do not waste this in cooking add to foods for flavor.

Almond

Delicate and useful in savory and sweet dishes and often used as a massage oil.

There are many health benefits in these oils but do remember they are high in calories so use in moderation.

Monosaturated oil particularly olive and rapeseed help to raise the good cholesterol (HDL) and contains vitamin E a natural anti-oxidant. Polyunsaturated fats provide us with the Omega 3 and 6. All oils should be fresh and stored in a cool dark place.

Pasta

I have great difficulty in advising the use of pasta, it is just wheat, water and sometimes egg depending on the type of pasta. Buckwheat is gluten free so has an advantage. I would not recommend using more than once a week and if you can use buckwheat, corn or rice pasta that would be preferable.

Noodles

Same advice as for pasta

Spices

There are many spices, all with health benefits as well as adding a great taste to your food. It is always best to buy fresh and in small amounts, pods or seeds rather than ground as the flavor will be retained.

I am going to list a few that you will probably want to use on the 30 day plan.

Allspice

Small berries with a sweet flavor. Can be added to marinades or in oatcakes for a different flavor. Sometimes added to curry for a sweeter taste. Grind before use. Great for the digestion and to avoid flatulence.

Cinnamon

These come in sticks or a ready ground powder. The sticks can be used in sweet or savory dishes but remove the stick before serving. If stewing apple or pear put a stick in whilst simmering slowly. Great for cleansing and anti-bacterial.

Caraway

These little seeds have an aniseed flavor which works well with sweet or savory dishes. Can be used whole or slightly crushed. Nice added to potato, cabbage and carrots for a twist in flavor. Good for digestion and flatulence.

Cardamon

The pods can be used whole or slightly crushed to release the full flavor. Works well in both savory and sweet dishes, often used in curry to bring a sweeter taste to the dish. Infused in hot rice or soya milk is a nice warm flavorsome drink. You can chew the seeds to freshen your breath. Calms digestion.

Cloves

These are mainly used in sweet dishes such as apple or pear. Use as cardamom but remove before serving. Long used as a cure for toothache for both its antiseptic and anesthetic qualities.

Nutmeg

Nutmeg is used in sweet dishes, can be added to porridge and also works well to liven up savory sauces. Buy the whole fruit and grate as required. Good for digestion.

Cayenne

A fiery spice which adds color and heat but not too much in the way of taste. It is from the capsicum family so you will be familiar which chilies and peppers. It is a digestive stimulant but anyone with a sensitive digestion should avoid this as it can aggravate the stomach.

Chilies

I have already said earlier that fresh are best so use a very little amount of the powder. Be careful if your digestive system is sensitive.

Coriander

This, together with cumin rate highly in curry making. The seeds have a different flavor than the fresh leaves. Grind the seeds as you need them for a quality flavor. Good for digestion

Cumin

Used in curry making but also works well with tomato based dishes. Slightly bitter taste. Use whole seeds and grind. Dry frying for 60 seconds enhances the flavor.

Fenugreek

Another popular spice used in curry making. A bitter taste, seeds are hard to grind. Good for digestion and cleansing.

Ginger

Where possible always use the ginger root as the flavor is far more satisfying than the powder. This is so versatile it can be used in soups, curries, stir fry, marinades, juicing and added to hot water for drinking. Great for the digestion and the immune system. The best way to handle this is to peel the root and freeze, when you need to use it pull it out of the freezer and grate. Or just peel and slice.

Lemon Grass

This comes in a long fibrous stalk, it has a citrus flavor and used in Thai cooking, adds a lovely flavor when used with coconut. Remove the woody outer layer, remove the root and crush or chop finely.

Galangal

Looks like ginger root. Prepare in the same way, good with curry, stir fry and Thai dishes.

Paprika

Milder than Cayenne, but still be aware if you have digestive problems.

Saffron

Very expensive if you buy a quality product but you only need a small amount. Adds a bitter sweet taste but often is used because it adds a lovely color to rice or other dishes. Good for calming the digestive system.

Tumeric

Used as an alternative to Saffron adds an earthy or peppery taste but also an interesting yellow to rice or other dishes. It has anti-bacterial and anti-fungal properties.

Vanilla

I recommend using this to flavor porridge but only buy the pod which you can infuse and remove to be used again, or pure essence.

You can also use it with fruits, soya or rice milk drinks.

This is not a complete list of spices or their benefits as we will go into this in full detail in the cookery book, DVD or the website. We will show you how to grind your own spices to make a curry paste, far superior to anything you purchase in a jar readymade and of course you can tailor it to your liking.

Fact File J
Vitamins & Minerals: Food Sources & Benefits
You will note a complete range of foods, please CHOOSE wisely!

VITAMIN	PURPOSE	WHERE FOUND
BIOFLAVANOIDS	Works with Vitamin C, antioxidant, antiviral and helps stabilize collagen matrix, anti-inflammatory properties. Deficiency can be linked with eczema, immune sluggishness, gum bleeding, glaucoma, heavy menstrual bleeding (with vitamin C), herpes, vaginitis, bruising.	Bilberry, citrus fruits, green tea, berries, legumes, parsley, red wine, strong colored fruits and vegetables, buckwheat.
CHOLINE	Important in normal nerve transmission, helps regulate liver and gallbladder. Deficiency can lead to fatty liver, high blood pressure, dementia, hemorrhaging, atherosclerosis, kidneys.	Lecithin, nuts, offal, egg yolk, wheat germ, brewer's yeast, pulses, soybeans, fish, beef, legumes, nuts.
FOLIC ACID	Necessary for growth and division of red blood cells, aids metabolism of proteins, also helps make RNA and DNA, aids transmission of genetic code. Deficiency can cause anemia, poor growth, poor memory, fatigue,	Alfalfa sprouts, chick peas, milk, yeasts, soya beans, cheese, nuts, lentils, sesame seeds, whole grains,

irritability, weakness, and problems in new-born, spin bifida.

avocado, salmon, dark green leafy vegetables, eggs, offal, wheat germ.

VITAMIN A (Retinol and betacarotene)

Necessary for growth and repair of body tissues, health of eyes, fights bacteria and infection, aids in bone, nerve and teeth formation. Beta carotene is best form, esp. during pregnancy. Deficiency can cause skin infection, scaly skin and scalp, poor hair, headaches, and impaired or dry eyes,

Spirulina, fish liver oils, liver, kidney, eggs, milk, butter, margarine, cream, cheese, carrots, sweet potatoes, squash, yellow and green fruits and vegetables.

VITAMIN B1 (Thiamine)

Needed for the release of energy from food, essential for digestion, nervous system, stress. Deficiency can result in tiredness, nausea, loss of appetite, depression, poor concentration, prickly legs, constipation, rapid heartbeat, and tingling hands.

Dried brewer's yeast, green vegetables, tomatoes, cauliflower, mushrooms, whole grains, brown rice, soya flour, oat flakes, offal, fish, poultry, legumes, nuts, molasses, and milk.

VITAMIN B2 (Riboflavin)	Aids in formation of antibodies and red blood cells, maintains cell respiration. Deficiency can cause cracks and sores on mouth, eczema or dermatitis, split nails, gritty eyes.	Liver, fish, milk, eggs, leafy green vegetables, bean sprouts, bamboo shoots, tomatoes, lean meat, fortified bread and cereals, egg yolks.
VITAMIN B3 (niacin)	Releases energy from food, balances blood sugar levels and lower cholesterol, helps maintain healthy skin, hair and the lining of organs such as nose and throat. Deficiency can cause digestive disturbances, sore mouth and gums, inflammation, dermatitis, diarrhea, dementia.	Yeast extract, whole wheat, fish, dried fruits, chicken liver, beef, milk, milk products, soya beans, mushrooms, squash, cauliflower, tomatoes,
VITAMIN B5 (Pantothenic acid)	Involved with the body's immune system, participates in the release of energy from carbohydrates, fats and protein. Deficiency can lead to vomiting, restlessness, blood and skin disorders, loss of appetite, digestive problems, respiratory infections, fatigue.	Meat, whole grains, wheat germ, pulses, organ meats, egg yolks, green vegetables, nuts, lentils, , avocados, strawberries, celery, tomatoes,

		squash, poultry, salmon, mushrooms,
VITAMIN B6 (Pyridoxine)	Helps make healthy red blood cells and regulates nervous system, anti-depressant, sex hormones PMT & menopause, works as a natural diuretic, amino acid metabolism. Deficiency can lead to split lips, inflammation of tongue and nerve endings, dermatitis, dandruff, water retention, muscle tremor or cramps, low energy,	Wheat germ, oats, soya, green & root vegetables, squash, bananas, cauliflower, mackerel, liver, nuts & seeds, rice, kidney beans, lentils, meats.
VITAMIN B12 (Cyanocobalamin)	Maintains healthy nervous system (myelin sheath), essential for the production of red blood cells. Deficiency can cause anemia and pernicious anemia, hair loss, nervousness, eczema, neuritis, energy loss, constipation, sore muscles, pale skin.	Spirulina, offal, sardines, oysters, tuna, mackerel, eggs, cheese, cottage cheese, full-fat milk, cheese, turkey, chicken.
VITAMIN C (Ascorbic acid)	Gives strength to blood vessels, will help provide resistance to infections, anti-oxidant, aids in absorption of iron, important for healthy skin, collagen maintenance, gums and blood vessels. Controls cholesterol and	Citrus fruit, guavas, berries, melons, parsley, green peppers, kale, horseradish, watercress, brussel sprouts,

activates folic acid. Deficiency can lead to nosebleeds, swollen or painful joints, easy bruising.

kale, potatoes, tomatoes, alfalfa seeds.

VITAMIN D (Cholecalciferol)

Helps body to absorb calcium and phosphorous, helps in treatment of conjunctivitis. Deficiency can cause softening of bones, poor teeth formation.

Cod liver oil, sardines, herrings, salmon, tuna, full-fat milk and dairy products, dark green leafy vegetables, cottage cheese, eggs.

VITAMIN E (Tocopherol)

Needed for muscle strength and hormone production, antioxidants; may prevent and dissolve blood clots. Deficiencies can lead to muscular wasting, rupture of red blood cells, lack of vitality & concentration, lethargy, apathy, infertility.

Wheat germ oil, avocados, seed oils/seeds/'seed' foods e.g. beans, almonds, nuts, spinach, wheat germ, cod liver oil, peanuts, soya sweet potatoes.

VITAMIN K

Essential for blood clotting, helps to prevent internal bleeding and hemorrhage, aids in reducing excessive menstrual flow. Deficiency can increase the tendency to hemorrhage.

Cauliflower, brussel sprouts, kelp, cabbage, spinach, broccoli, peas, wholegrain cereals, egg yolk, fish liver oil, potatoes, beans, tomatoes.

BIOTIN	Essential for breaking down and metabolizing fats in the body, glucose activity, important for healthy skin tissues. Deficiency can result in muscle pain, dermatitis, depression, extreme exhaustion.	Baker's yeast, liver, kidney, brown rice, mushrooms ,wheat germ, oats, eggs, cauliflower, whole meal bread, mackerel, sardines, milk.
BORON	Helps with vitamin D activity, bone-strengthening, helps prevent or relieve osteoporosis and arthritis, acts as gate-keeper for estrogen. Deficiency may be associated with postmenopausal bone loss.	Root vegetables, alfalfa, cabbage, peas, fruits and vegetables generally. Cider, wine & beer.
CALCIUM	For strong teeth and healthy bones, neutralizes acid in body, helps to maintain nerve and muscle function, cholesterol levels and regular heart beat rhythm. Works closely with Magnesium and Vitamin D. Deficiency can cause muscle cramps, arthritis, rickets, bone loss, teeth decay, and high	Cheddar cheese, skimmed milk, seeds, tofu, almonds, fish with bones, prunes, sardines, green & root vegetables, yoghurt, dried

blood pressure.

cooked beans.

CHROMIUM

Essential for proper utilization of carbohydrates and glucose, reducing diabetic and hypoglycemic tendencies, heart function. Deficiency can cause mental confusion, irritability, depression, learning difficulties cold sweats, dizziness, need for food, excessive sleep, thirst, sweet cravings

Meat, kidney, liver, milk, raisins, clams, yeast, egg yolk, wholegrain products, cheese, butter, chicken, parsnips, green peppers, potatoes, apples.

COBALT

Helps with vitamin B12 production, red blood cell formation, and enzyme activation. Deficiency is very rare; can be linked with anemia, weakness, numbness, balance, paleness, and poor blood symptoms.

Vegetable greens, cabbage, figs, shellfish, offal, buckwheat, green leafy vegetables & fruit, meat, eggs.

COPPER

Helps formation of red blood cells, co-factor for many enzymes, skin healing, and nerve impulses in brain, essential for the utilization of vitamin C. Deficiencies include general weakness, prominent veins, diarrhea, water retention, brittle bones, loss of taste,

Shellfish, offal, baker's yeast, crab, oats, whole meal bread, lentils, olives, nuts, raisins.

IODINE

Regulates energy and rate of metabolism especially involved

Iodized salts, seafood, kelp,

with the thyroid, promotes growth, and helps with dieting by burning excess fat. Deficiency leads to dry skin and hair, loss of physical and mental vigor, goiter, weight gain, coarse skin

seaweed, potatoes, carrots, onions, garlic, berries, and wholegrain cereals.

IRON

Essential for making red blood cells and oxygen uptake, necessary for energy and vitality, promotes resistance to disease. Deficiency can lead to poor vision, tiredness, and anemia, indigestion, tingling in fingers and toes, poor appetite, brittle nails, sensitivity to cold.

Molasses, spirulina, kelp, cooked dried beans, seafood, nuts, seeds, whole meal bread, spinach, offal, red meat, eggs, dried apricots, dried figs, parsley.

Magnesium

Known as an anti-stress mineral, keeps the circulatory system, bones, teeth, nerves and muscles healthy, can help indigestion. Deficiency can result in insomnia, nervousness, tremors, depression, tiredness, muscle cramps, weakness, high blood pressure, confusion.

Nuts (esp. cashew), seeds, baker's yeast, brown rice, whole meal bread and pasta, green leafy vegetables, shrimps, crab, bananas, beans, peas.

MANGANESE

Necessary for normal skeletal

Berries,

development, enzyme activator, improves memory, reduces nervous irritability, insulin production. Deficiency can lead to convulsions, blindness and deafness in infants, diabetes, muscle twitching, dizziness, sore knees & joint pains

pineapple, nuts, okra, endive, grapes, lettuce, lima beans, oats, beetroot, celery.

MOLYBDENUM

Aids with mobilization of iron from liver reserves and helps rid the body of protein breakdown, e.g. uric acid, helps prevent tooth decay and impotence. Deficiency can result in premature ageing, irregular heartbeat, irritability, and dental caries.

Tomatoes, whole-wheat products, wheat germ, eggs, offal, soya, lentils, beans, rye, spinach, pork, lamb...

POTASSIUM

Works to control activity of heart muscles, nervous systems and kidneys, keeps tissues in good tone. Enables nutrients & waste to move in & out of cells, maintains fluid balance, relaxes muscle, aids secretion of insulin for blood sugar control, stimulates gut movements to encourage elimination. Deficiency can result in poor reflexes, constipation, liver disorders, rapid/irregular heartbeat, irritability, nausea, vomiting, diarrhea, swollen

All foods, esp. watercress, molasses, dried fruit, nuts, vegetables, bananas, potatoes, red peppers, parsley, mushrooms, endive, cabbage, celery, cauliflower, pumpkin, courgettes,

	abdomen, cellulite, low blood pressure, confusion, mental clarity	radishes.
SELENIUM	Anti-oxidant. Helps to maintains a healthy liver, also vital as an antioxidant, helps keep youthful elasticity in tissues, hair, eyes & skin, boosts immune system, reduces inflammation, helps vitamin E action, reproductive system. Deficiency can result in hair loss, low resistance to disease, premature stamina/aging loss, high blood pressure, family history of cancer,	Organ meats, muscle meats, fish and shellfish, cottage cheese, cabbage, courgettes, whole meal bread, cheddar cheese, carrots, turnip, mushrooms.
SILICON	Small but vital part of all connective tissues, bones, blood vessels and cartilage, helps strengthens skin, hair and nails. Deficiency can lead to weakened or rough skin tissue.	Root vegetables, brown rice, hard drinking water, some mineral waters, oatmeal, green leafy vegetables.
SODIUM	Maintains normal fluid levels in cells, maintains health of the nervous, muscular, blood and lymph systems. **Often excessive in diets.** Deficiency very rare; can cause nausea, loss of appetite, intestinal gas, dizziness, heat exhaustion, low blood	Olives, yeast extract, sauerkraut, shrimps, miso, beetroot, celery, cabbage, cottage cheese, red kidney beans,

pressure, rapid pulse, mental apathy, muscle cramps, nausea, vomiting, headache.

bacon, salami, tinned ham, smoked ham, stilton, and many processed foods.

SULPHUR

Helps create healthy, supple skin, assists the liver, tones up the whole system, and helps fight bacterial infections. Deficiency (rare) can cause sluggishness and fatigue.

Shellfish, beef, eggs, chicken, pork, dried peaches, pulses, peas, fish, cabbage, dried beans, garlic, mustard powder.

VANADIUM

Helpful for bone, cartilage and tooth development, insulin action, helps in preventing heart attacks. Possible lowering of cholesterol.

Shellfish, parsley, dill, nuts, wholegrain cereals, mushrooms, kelp, alfalfa.

ZINC

Aids in healing process, bone growth, controls hormone messengers from testes & ovaries, aids ability to cope with stress, bones, hair, energy, blood sugar levels (insulin), and liver function. Deficiency can result in diabetes, loss of taste/appetite and hair, eczema, stretch marks (along with

Brewer's yeast, liver, lamb, nuts, seafood (esp. oysters), cheese, meat, lentils, whole grains, seeds, nuts, eggs, ginger root.

Vitamin E), white spots on nails,
loss of taste and smell,
depression, loss of appetite.

Fact File K
Choosing To Eat Meat

Contrary to popular belief we do not need to eat these foods to get our full   requirement of protein. It does take a little more thought to put it all together but you really don't need that slab of flesh on your plate or in that bun with onions and fries.

So what about our history of meat eating and why do we have teeth that can chew. There is many a debate as to whether or not our teeth were designed to chew meat or perhaps chew the tougher vegetables and perhaps more raw food.

The digestive system, in my view, gives us a bit of a clue. Digestion begins in the mouth when you are chewing; the enzymes that are present are those which start to process carbohydrates, NOT protein, our digestive system is a very long tube with compartments doing specific jobs. (see Digestive System in Chapter 3 for more explanation on this) not like that of a typical carnivore such as, say a dog, who has no enzymes in its saliva, and does not chew food, merely tears it into pieces big enough to swallow, the food then hits the stomach where a highly acidic environment breaks down the protein.

It is a certainty that even if early man ate meat he would have been in a contest with the animal kingdom to get his share on the day. Humans have evolved and become meat eaters, but was that choice or greed? It was considered that man who ate grains was a peasant while the man who ate flesh was a king. Maybe it really is all about image!

There are far more important reasons not to choose meat, the overuse of growth hormones in the food chain. Antibiotics are used extensively to not only help to prevent disease because of poor husbandry due to overcrowding but feeding lower but regular doses of disease fighting antibiotics has been found to increase the growth of the animal Have you ever noticed how cattle seem to be bigger than they used to be?

And of course we could look at the way animals are slaughtered it is appalling. If anyone ever bothers to check this out I feel it would seriously affect what you choose to eat. I say, don't eat anything with a face on it!

Anyway I am not going to delve too deeply into the politics of this as there are many others who have done so. This book is about choices and I want you to be able to make those.

Growth Hormones

- rBGH bovine growth hormones are injected into cattle to make them grow faster and bigger

Antibiotics

- These are being used to combat the higher incidence of mastitis in cows which is a severe infection of the udder due to massive more milk production caused by the use of rBGH
- They are used in a milder form in cattle feed regularly to promote growth and with overstocking it helps to reduce disease.

Other vaccines that are being used, considered or trialed are those for foot and mouth disease, bovine TB and mad cow disease. What a choice.

All of this is happening because we have this massive market for meat production which means that cattle are reared on grain which does not suit their digestive system as they are designed to eat and digest grass but it does mean they can all be crowded in pens and fed without the need for grass, of course where they would normally be grazing, the grain is being grown as there will be more yield per hectare than grazing would give to the animal. And of course it is far easier to add chemicals and antibiotics to grain.

Chickens which are reared for their flesh are packed by the thousands into sheds where they are fed masses of antibiotics and drugs to keep them alive in such appalling conditions that otherwise they would not survive. The antibiotics, as well as preventing disease, encourage chickens to grow very quickly and to such a large size they cannot even stand up. Notice the difference in size between and organic chicken and a mass reared one. And what about the eggs...if you are going to eat any of this, choose organic!

If you ate less flesh, no processed meat such as burgers, luncheon meat, ready meat meals, then the whole environment would change as there would be less forced farming methods. Remember, I am not saying don't eat meat. But, hopefully you will, by the end of this book, choose more wisely for your health. This is just the tip of the iceberg; if you're interested in more information, please visit my website www.TrishaStewart.com

Fact File L

The Glycaemic Index

High GI
70 plus

Medium GI
56 - 69

Low GI
1 - 55

The GI or glycaemic index is a system of measuring how different carbohydrate rich foods act on blood sugar levels. A rule of thumb is anything 55 or below because it will act slower therefore sustaining the blood sugar levels.

The GL or glycaemic load is another way of measuring. It lets us know the quality of the carbohydrate. For instance the carbohydrate of the watermelon has a high GI but there is not a lot of carbohydrate in the watermelon so the actual load or GL on the body is low. This means then that the watermelon will spike you up fairly quickly but it will not add too much carbohydrate into your diet.

We'll show more of this on the website as it's another way of working with your food. I'm not too keen on counting either calories or GI/GL but if you're not well, suffering from Diabetes or have other reasons to know what your GI/GL is then it's a good way of monitoring your intake and knowing about both is very useful.

Glycaemic Index (foods selected are based around what we are doing over the 30 days and of course beyond but a more comprehensive index will be available on the website)

Food	grams	GI	GL
Whole oats	250	51	11
Pot Barley	150	25	11
Buckwheat	150	54	16
Polenta	150	69	9
Millet	150	71	25
Wholegrain Rice	150	55	18
Rice Noodles	180	61	23
Rice Cakes	25	78	17
Quinoa			
Butter beans	150	31	6
Black-eyed beans	150	42	13
Chick peas	150	28	8
Haricot beans	150	38	12
Red Kidney beans	150	28	7
Lentils	150	30	5
Pinto beans	150	39	10
Soya beans	150	18	1
Broad beans	80	79	9
Peas	80	48	3
Pumpkin	80	75	3
Sweetcorn	80	54	9
Carrots	80	47	3
Potatoes (white)	150	88	16 boiled
		85	26 baked
		75	22 fries
		91	18 mashed
Sweet Potato	150	44	11
Swede	150	72	7
Apple	120	38	6
Apricot	120	57	5
Banana	120	52	12
Grapes	120	49	9
Kiwi	120	53	6

Food	grams	GI	GL
Orange	120	42	5
Peach	120	42	5
Pears	120	38	4
Plum	120	39	5
Strawberries	120	40	1
Pineapple	120	66	6
Mango	120	51	8
Grapefruit	120	25	3
Cherries	120	22	3
Watermelon	120	72	4
Hummus	30	6	0
Cashew Nuts	50	22	3

Fact File M
Sugar by Any Other Name Is Still Sugar

1. **Brown sugar (sucrose)**
Sugar crystals contained in a molasses syrup.

2. **Corn syrup (glucose)**
Made from cornstarch.

3. **Demerara Sugar (sucrose)**
A light brown sugar with large golden crystals which are slightly sticky.

4. **Dextrose (glucose)**
Commonly known as corn sugar and grape sugar

5. **Free Flowing Brown Sugars (sucrose)**
These sugars are fine, powder-like brown sugars that are much like white sugar.

6. **Fructose**
Naturally occurring sugar found in fruit and honey.

7. **Galactose**
Sugar found linked to glucose to form lactose, or milk sugar.

8. **Glucose**
Also called dextrose. Most of the carbohydrates you eat are converted to glucose in the body.

9. **High Fructose Corn Syrup**
Derived from cornstarch, usually a combination of 55 percent fructose and 45 percent sucrose. Is HIGHLY

refined and used a lot in readymade products, particularly junk food. It is treated with an enzyme that converts glucose to fructose, this results in a very sweet product. Used in soft drinks, baked goods, jelly, syrups, fruits and desserts.

10. **Honey (fructose and glucose)**
Made by bees from the nectar collected from flowers and stored in nests or hives as food.

11. **Lactose (glucose and galactose)**
Sugar found in milk and milk products.

12. **Maltose**
Also called malt sugar. Used in the fermentation of alcohol by converting starch to sugar. The primary sugar in beer.

13. **Maple syrup (sucrose)**
A concentrated sucrose solution made from mature sugar maple tree sap.

14. **Molasses**
Thick syrup left after making sugar from sugar cane. Brown in color with a high sugar concentration.

15. **Muscovado or Barbados Sugar (sucrose)**
A very dark brown sugar which has a particularly strong molasses flavor.

16. **Powdered or confectioner's sugar**
Ground common sugar.

17. **Sucrose**
Commonly called cane sugar or table sugar.

18. **Sugar (granulated)**

Refined cane or beet sugar; 100 percent sucrose.

19. **Turbinado sugar**

Raw sugar that has been partially refined and washed.

Fact File N

The Truth about Artificial Sweeteners

For too long we've been told that using sugar substitutes...artificial sweeteners...that we're helping 'the battle of the bulge'. It's true that you take in fewer calories, and that is a positive thing. However, the down side to using artificial sweetener greatly outweighs the up side. First, it's been shown that many sugar substitutes cause your body to react in the same way as if you were eating real sugar. What that means is your blood sugar or glucose levels still rise and fall when these products enter your body. It also means you're doing NOTHING to help alleviate your craving for sugar. Your body will want more of whatever sweetener you give it (outside of a few natural products that do NOT affect your blood sugar).

But perhaps even worse is the harmful impact these artificial sweeteners can have on your body. The latest villain in the sugar substitute game is aspartame. It is the technical name for several brand name sweeteners including NutraSweet, Equal, Spoonful, and Equal-Measure.

Here's a partial list of the maladies associated with aspartame:

Headaches/migraines, dizziness, seizures, nausea, numbness, muscle spasms,   weight gain, rashes, depression, fatigue, irritability, tachycardia, insomnia, vision problems, hearing loss, heart palpitations, breathing difficulties, anxiety attacks, slurred speech, loss of taste, tinnitus, vertigo, memory loss, and joint pain.

And, it's been known to trigger or worsen brain tumors, multiple sclerosis, epilepsy, chronic fatigue syndrome, Parkinson's disease, Alzheimer's, mental retardation, lymphoma, birth defects, fibromyalgia, and diabetes.

And, although use of this product has been linked to everything from memory loss to brain tumors...it's still listed as a 'safe' food additive! Personally, I feel it is one of the most dangerous substances on the market that is added to foods. There are a number of great articles and books written on this subject, so I won't try to go into it all here. But, if you want more information on aspartame or other artificial sweeteners, visit my website: www.TrishaStewart.com. If you don't find what you're looking for...send me an email and I'll be sure the information is made available.

Fact File O
Heavy Metals – Sources & Symptoms

Aluminum

Sources: Aluminum foil, antacids, aspirin, dust, auto exhaust, treated water, vanilla powder, nasal spray, milk products, salt, commercially-raised beef, tobacco smoke, antiperspirants, bleached flour, cans, animal feed, ceramics and commercial cheese

Symptoms and Diseases: Flatulence, headaches, dry skin, weak and aching muscles, senility, spleen pain, stomach pain, liver dysfunction, kidney dysfunction, neuromuscular disorders, osteomalacia, colitis, anemia, Alzheimer's disease, amyotrophic lateral sclerosis, hemolysis, leukocytosis, porphyria, heartburn, memory loss, numbness, paralysis, Parkinson's disease, excessive perspiration, leg twitching, cavities, colds, behavioral problems and constipation.

Arsenic

Sources: Coal combustion, paints, rat poisoning, beer, pesticides, table salt, seafood from coastal waters (oysters, shrimp, muscles), fungicides, drinking water and wood preservatives.

Symptoms and Diseases: Enzyme inhibitor, anorexia, diarrhea, nausea, vomiting, chronic anemia, drowsiness, dermatitis, stomatitis, liver dysfunction, hair loss, headache, vertigo, fever, stupor, herpes, jaundice, fluid loss, throat constriction, spasms, respiratory tract infection, garlicky odor to breath or stool, keritosis, pallor and goiter.

Cadmium

Sources: Tap water, fungicides, marijuana, processed meat, rubber, seafood (cod, haddock, oyster, tuna), sewage, tobacco, colas (especially from vending machines), tools, welding material, evaporated milk, airborne industrial contaminants, batteries, instant coffee, incineration of tires/rubber/plastic, refined grains, soft water, galvanized pipes, dental alloys, candy, ceramics, electroplating fertilizers, paints, motor oil and motor exhaust.

Symptoms and Diseases: Alopecia, anemia, arthritis, cancer, lung disease, cerebral hemorrhage, cirrhosis of the liver, enlarged heart, diabetes, emphysema, hypoglycemia, hypertension, impotence, infertility, kidney disease, learning disorders, migraines, inflammation, renal disease, osteoporosis, schizophrenia, strokes, vascular disease, high cholesterol, growth is impaired and cardiovascular disease,

Copper

Sources: Copper cookware, copper pipes, dental alloys, fungicides, ice makers, industrial emissions, swimming pools, shellfish, perch, bluefish, lobster, walnuts, almonds, soybeans, wheat germ, yeast, beer, chocolate, corn oil, gelatin, liver, lamb, mushrooms, avocados and birth control pills.

Symptoms and Diseases: Acne, allergies, alopecia, insomnia, nausea, spaciness, tooth decay, strokes, PMS, yeast infections, urinary tract infections, mood swings, kidney disorders, depression, cystic fibrosis, arthritis, anxiety, anorexia, multiple sclerosis, inflammation, pancreatic dysfunction, vitamin deficiencies, paranoia, migraines, libido decreased, nervousness, osteoporosis, senility, stuttering, phobias, diabetes, autism and estrogen dominance.

Iron

Sources: Iron cookware, iron pipes, drinking water, welding, shellfish, soybeans, liver, kidneys, beef, nuts, legumes, sunflower seeds, bran, bone meal, wheat germ, whole grain, molasses, and yeast.

Symptoms and Diseases: Anger and other emotional disorders, birth defects, constipation, diabetes, insomnia, high blood pressure, arthritis, cancer, cirrhosis of the liver, schizophrenia, myasthenia gravis, nausea, pancreas damage, headaches, Parkinson's disease, scurvy, shortness of breath, hepatitis, dizziness, heart failure.

Lead

Sources: Ash, auto exhaust, cigarette smoke, coal combustion, colored inks, pesticides, rainwater, food cans with lead solder sealing, toothpaste, wine, manufacturing batteries, cosmetics, hair dyes, lead pipes, liver, glazed ceramics, pencils, lead-based paint and industrial emissions.

Symptoms and Diseases: Abdominal pain, ADD, adrenal insufficiency, allergies, anemia, anxiety, arthritis, blindness, cardiovascular disease, autism, colic, constipation, convulsions, depression, dyslexia, epilepsy, fatigue, gout, hallucinations, headaches, hostility, hyperactivity, hypertension, hypothyroidism, impotence, liver dysfunction, hyperkinesis, mental retardation, mood swings, menstrual problems, muscular dystrophy, multiple sclerosis, nephritis, nightmares, nausea, numbness, Parkinson's disease, poor concentration, psychosis, renal dysfunction, restlessness, schizophrenia, seizures, stillbirths, tooth decay, vertigo and unexplained weight loss.

Mercury

Sources: Dental amalgam, tuna fish, swordfish, felt, algaecides, floor waxes, adhesives, fabric softeners, chlorine production, contact lens solution, preparation H, diuretics, Mercurochrome, Merthiolate and some childhood vaccines.

Symptoms and Diseases: Adrenal gland dysfunction, anorexia, birth defects, brain damage, depression, dermatitis, dizziness, fatigue, hearing loss, hyperactivity, insomnia, kidney damage, memory loss, migraines, mood swings, nervousness, pain in limbs, skin rashes, schizophrenia, thyroid dysfunction and peripheral vision loss.

Nickel

Sources: Peanut butter, hydrogenated vegetable oils, margarine, imitation whip creams, kelp, oysters, herring, nickel plating, cigarette smoking, tea, batteries, wire and electrical parts.

Symptoms and Diseases: Hemorrhages, malaise, low blood pressure, kidney dysfunction, nausea, vomiting, heart attack, oral cancer, and intestinal cancer.

Tin

Sources: Tin coated cans of fruits and vegetables, processed foods and industrial waste.

Symptoms and Diseases: Headaches, vomiting, diarrhea, abdominal cramping, abdominal bloating, nausea, fever, hyperglycemia, vision changes, liver pain, and ataxia.

Fact File P

Mold: How to Handle & Avoid Moldy Food

Just being more aware that mold is out there should make you diligent enough to keep mold free. A great idea for some 'mold-prone' items is to buy in small amounts and use the food quickly...plan ahead. However, if you do discover any moldy food, please keep in mind:

- Don't sniff the moldy item. This can cause respiratory trouble.
- If food is covered with mold, discard it. Wrap it up and dispose in a covered trash can that children and animals can't get into.
- Clean the refrigerator or pantry at the spot where the food was stored.
- Check nearby items the moldy food might have touched. Mold spreads quickly in fruits and vegetables.

So, here are a few tips – especially if you've recently discovered some moldy food in your refrigerator:

- Clean the inside of the refrigerator every few months with 1 tablespoon of baking soda dissolved in a liter or so of water. Rinse with clear water and dry. Scrub visible mold (usually black) on rubber casings using 3 teaspoons of washing soda in a liter or so of water.

- Keep dishcloths, towels, sponges, and mops clean and fresh. A musty smell means they're spreading mold around. Discard items you can't clean or launder.
- Keep the humidity level in the house below 40%.

What about the food you buy? How long has it been sitting on the shelf or in that display case? Here are a few tips for mold-free shopping, cooking and serving:

- Examine food well before you buy it. Check food in glass jars, look at the stem areas on fresh produce, and avoid bruised produce. Do not accept these foods where you shop.
- And, for those carnivores out there, I have to say this. Fresh meat and poultry are usually mold free, but cured and cooked meats may not be. Examine them carefully. Exceptions: Some salamis have a characteristic thin, white mold coating. they shouldn't show any other mold. Dry-cured country hams normally have surface mold that must be scrubbed off before cooking.
- Molds can thrive in high-acid foods like jams, jellies, pickles, fruit, and tomatoes. But these microscopic fungi are easily destroyed by heat processing high-acid foods at a temperature of 212 °F in a boiling water

pan   for   the   recommended   length   of   time.

- When serving food, keep it covered to prevent exposure to mold spores in the air. Use plastic wrap to cover foods you want to stay moist - fresh or cut fruits and vegetables, and green and mixed salads.

- Empty opened cans of perishable foods into clean storage containers and refrigerate them promptly.

- Don't leave any perishables out of the refrigerator for more than 2 hours.

- Use leftovers within 3 to 4 days so mold doesn't have a chance to grow.

Afterword

So, where do you go from here?

I hope you have enjoyed reading this book and, more importantly, that you have achieved the Healthy Tartness you've worked so hard to achieve. I've written this book so you can always refer to it and work through the steps time and time again...so you can always maintain your health and vitality.

And, you now have the experience to "tune in" to your body, carefully listening to its requirements. You're no longer listening to what your head is saying...because those old habits are what made you unhealthy in the first place. Those old habits are now buried in the long distant past.

What you have now is a permanent lifestyle in which you can enjoy yourself, have fun and have all the vitality in the world to be able to do whatever you desire, while being totally aware of what you're eating and why...when to fuel up or when you need to cut back. The basics here will never change. This way of eating is something that will serve you well for the rest of your life. There is nothing "faddy" about this book, no "quick fixes" as you have read, several times.

I'm sure you'll want you to share your new found health with your friends and family. I want that too. That's why I'm creating the following books:

You don't have to be a Superman to be a Healthy Dude
The Healthy Dude Book is a great guide for any man in your life that speaks to the male side of health, food and fitness. It covers everything from how to develop a real six-pack to why he might want to put down the "other" six-pack.

Get Your 'Healthy' Groove On! With Healthy Idol
Healthy Idol is a book written for those teens to twenties who want to be the best they can be and avoid the pitfalls along the way. With advice on eating right, avoiding excess, getting in shape and setting goals, Healthy Idol is the 'must have' guide to Health, Success and Physical Wellbeing.

You don't have to be a little health nut to be a Healthy Pumpkin
This is the book for those little darlings twelve and under who need the right information...not the latest fad...in order to grow big, strong and healthy. This is a resource you can trust to help children build a healthy mind set and a healthy body.

Healthy Bunch Cook Book
A cookbook for Healthy Tarts, Dudes and Pumpkins

This cookbook will show you how to cook tasty meals, have healthy lunch boxes and whip up satisfying snacks every day for the rest of your life. Whether you're a gourmet cook or a beginner in the kitchen...you'll love the variety and easy to follow recipes!

Also look out for Christin McDowell's new book 'Healthy Fitness Central'. It's a complete workout and fitness book designed for all ages and levels of fitness.

Don't forget that the Trisha Stewart team is always available to you. Our 24/7 online support provides useful tips, articles and in-depth information on your particular health issues. Plus you can always 'ask-the-expert' for whatever questions come to mind. Visit us at www.TrishaStewart.com.

Thank you for reading this book. I am grateful to be a part of your health journey and I want you to have the best health ever...so keep working at it!